Fine thanks mate

Fine thanks mate

JOHN 'BOMBER' PEARD
League, Life and Second Chances

JOHN PEARD
with Larry Writer

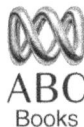

ABC
Books

Published by ABC Books for the
AUSTRALIAN BROADCASTING CORPORATION
GPO Box 9994 Sydney NSW 2001

First published in April 2007

ISBN 978 0 7333 2103 0

All pictures, unless those credited otherwise, are from John's personal
and family collections. Every effort has been made to establish the
copyright holder of those images that remain uncredited. The publishers
would be pleased to hear from the copyright holder/photographer to
rectify any omissions in future printings of this book.

*photography: (front cover) John Peard today (copyright Katrina Cook)
and in action at the 1975 semi-final, Saints vs Easts, at the SCG
(copyright Newspix/News Ltd). (back cover, left) The premiership-
winning Eastern Suburbs team of 1974, with John Peard in the back
row on the left. (right) Some serious footy talent visit a recovering
John in hospital.*

*The Bomber career stats prepared by Terry Liberopoulos, Rugby League Review
Cover and internals designed by Luke Causby/Blue Cork
Set in 11.5/18 pt Sabon by Kirby Jones*

To Mum and Dad
with love and thanks

ACKNOWLEDGEMENTS

Many authors say that without certain people their book could never have been written, but in my case, recovering from my stroke, it's 100 per cent true. Without the kindness and inspiration of the following people I could never have told my story.

So thank you from the bottom of my heart. To Mum and Dad, gone now but always in my thoughts. To my wife and best friend Chris. To my daughters Amanda and Johanna and their families. To my siblings Margaret (and her husband Peter Moscatt who ensured I never went hungry), Diane and Geoff and their families. To Jo Richards, Peter and Courtney Cruikshank, Graham Bowen, Greg Cummins, John Quayle, Arthur Beetson, Jack Gibson, Keiran Speed, Johnny Mayes, Fred Pagano, Bob McMillan, Dr Phil Dwyer, Kim Mitric, Larry Gaffney, Johnny Chisholm, and all my rugby league and other sporting friends who have enriched my life and whose names and exploits appear in this book. To Ron Coote, Jim Hall and Max Brown and all the wonderful Men of League. To Deanne and Rebecca, who got me through rehab, and all the staff at

Sutherland District Hospital. To everyone who reached out to help me and spoke encouraging words that have helped see me through the dark times in the months after my stroke, and to those who continue to do so today. To everyone who enjoyed seeing me play rugby league and who has laughed at my jokes, and every comedian whose jokes I've borrowed. To everyone I've forgotten to thank, thank you. And thanks, too, to Larry Writer who helped me to turn my memories, musings and beliefs into words on a page.

John Peard
Caringbah
February 6, 2007

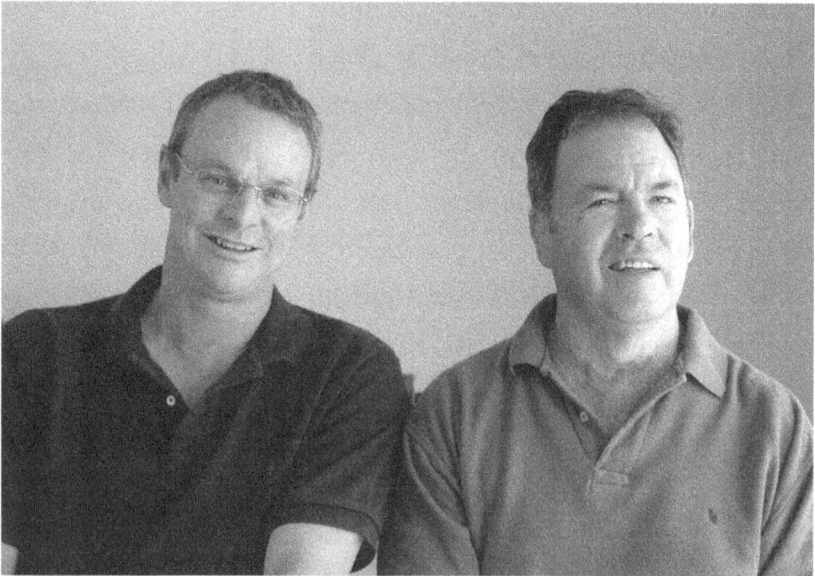

CONTENTS

FOREWORD

The Bomber

By John Quayle, team-mate, friend and former
chief executive of the Australian Rugby League

John Peard has been inspiring me all his life.

The first time was way back in 1968. I was a kid from the
bush who'd joined the Eastern Suburbs Roosters. John was a
promising local junior battling to get back into grade after a
year out of football thanks to glandular fever. Jack Gibson was
the coach and he wasn't about to do anybody any favours. To
regain his position as a graded player, let alone first grader, John
had to start from scratch and take part in a series of park trials
in front of the club selectors over a period of some weeks. He

was right behind the eight ball, he'd lost nearly twenty kilos and spent much of the past year in bed. But he was determined to make it. He knuckled down, played his heart out and trained every day, running laps, lifting weights, working on his skills.

It was so clear to us all that he had immense talent, but he dutifully battled on, playing those qualifying trials with the intensity of grand finals.

At that point, when his career was touch and go, I remember him telling me, 'Don't you worry, Jack. I'll make it.'

And he did.

When the season started, John was the Roosters' first-grade five-eighth. His illustrious career with Easts, St George, Parramatta and Australia was under way. John's passion and will to succeed astonished me. If I needed a role model, I'd found one.

He was a complete five-eighth. Not as brilliant a player perhaps as Raper, Gasnier or Langlands, and he was small, but he made up for all that by working harder to be great. He was a consummate linkman in attack, a punishing defender despite his size, and of course he was the Bomber – exponent of the most deadly and accurate up-and-under the game of rugby league had ever seen, which terrorised opposition teams for years and led to scores of tries for Russell Fairfax, Ian Schubert, Mark Harris, Ray Price, Mick Cronin and other greats of his era. The bomb didn't just happen. It was the end result of countless hours of practice at training and in a park near John's home.

John was a valuable member of any team. And not just for his footballing skills. He was (and remains) a nice man, a decent bloke, a staunch friend, who had the great gift of making people laugh. His quick-as-lightning quips and spot-on impersonations of Paul Hogan, Frank Hyde and Ken Howard were side-splittingly funny. He always had a smile on his face. No one enjoyed the great Australian way of life, typified by footy, the surf, a beer, a bet and good friends, more than Peardy.

John and I were both selected in the 1975 Australian World Series team to tour the United Kingdom and France. The bond we shared grew stronger through the ups and downs of our campaign. I saw at close hand the dedication of the man, how hard he trained, how he never cut a corner in his effort to be the best player he could be. In John's luggage was a heavy iron boot. He had a bad knee and before and after training he would put that boot on and sweat and strain through a gruelling series of knee lifts. It had taken him almost his whole career to achieve his childhood dream and make the Australian side, and he wasn't going to let the chance pass him by.

The match against Wales was a wild and woolly affair. With Arthur Beetson, George Piggins and Tom Raudonikis on our team and Jim Mills, Kel Coslett and Tony Fisher on theirs, this wasn't so much a football game, as a chance to see who could whack his opponent the hardest. I was a casualty of the mayhem. Jim Mills crunched me and dislocated my shoulder. At the team hotel in Wales the night after the game I was faced with the decision: to go home, or to continue in the Australian party, even though I'd be unable to play. John took me aside and quietly made me understand that the chance to be part of an Australian squad is a rare honour. I stayed with the team, with my right arm strapped to my body for the next three weeks.

Our team-mate John Brass was my official room-mate and Tom Raudonikis offered to look after me, but John would have none of it. 'He can room with me. He's going to need some special care. I'll make sure he's comfortable and has everything he needs,' he promised.

The first night in France after we'd beaten Wales, there was a celebration downstairs in the hotel bar. John said he'd get my dinner and bring it straight back. Eight hours later he still hadn't appeared. I was starving and unable even to call the bar – because I knew that's where he'd be – on the hotel room phone. Finally Tommy said to John, 'How's the Canon?' – that was my nickname. John did a double take: 'I've forgotten all about him!' I forgave him, of course, and he took perfect care of me from then on.

When John returned home from the tour, he left the Roosters. They were worried that he was getting on in years and that injuries were beginning to plague him. Parramatta had no such qualms. Coach Terry Fearnley knew what John was capable of, and I, who had joined Parramatta for season 1976, was delighted to play alongside him again. Peardy was exactly what the up-and-coming Eels needed. Unfortunately, my bad shoulder never came right and I retired midway through the year. It would have been a privilege joining Ray Price to chase down John's pinpoint bombs, but it wasn't to be.

John too – as we all must – retired from the game in 1979 and, needing an outlet for his love of rugby league and great tactical brain, he became a coach at Parramatta, Penrith and for New South Wales in the 1988 State of Origin. As chief executive of the Australian Rugby League I had no hesitation in giving him my full support for the prestigious job of coaching his state. John wasn't as successful as he would have wanted to be, but he can never be accused of not giving coaching his all. He knows no other way. Many New South Wales players told me that being coached by John Peard, with his superb football knowledge and tireless work ethic, made them far better footballers than before. He won their deep and abiding respect.

When John bowed out of coaching, he turned his talent to being an inspirational speaker and stand-up comedian. He travelled throughout Australia, entertaining audiences with his wisdom and hilarious jokes, delivered in his trademark dry-as-dust Aussie vernacular. He appeared at clubs, pubs and charity events, and would always waive his fee for a worthy cause.

Through his forties and fifties, John was the picture of health and vitality. He remained trim and strong. He was a man who refused to accept that he was no longer twenty-one. Wherever there was enjoyment and laughter, there'd be John. He seemed the least likely candidate to be laid low by serious illness.

I was in Athens in June 2002, advising on the upcoming Olympic Games, when my wife phoned to tell me that John had had a severe stroke. I couldn't believe it. Not John Peard, the man who was still training at age fifty-seven, still running, swimming and lifting weights. But it was true. I called John's wife, Chris. She told me that John might not survive.

Having known him so long and so well, I was in no doubt that if mental strength, determination and an ability and willingness to put in the hard work had anything to do with it, the odds for survival were with him. And slowly, surely, his condition improved.

Back in Australia I visited John at Sutherland Hospital where, characteristically, he was throwing himself into his rehabilitation. I still get emotional today when I conjure up the image of John, his body twisted and disabled, struggling with enormous difficulty to walk with the aid of a heavy frame. This was a man who knew he had been given a second chance at life and he wasn't going to waste it. Death or – perhaps worse for a man like John – life in a wheelchair wasn't an option.

Through many months of gruelling rehabilitation therapy and thanks to the kindness of loved ones such as his loving wife Chris and daughters Johanna and Amanda, and some incredible mates, John's condition slowly improved. Although his left side was terribly damaged by his stroke, he gradually taught himself to walk again, to think, to tie his laces, shower and make a cup of tea. Movement returned and so did his smile.

Today, John is still not out of the woods. Every day is a battle to live life in a way that most of us take for granted. Yet he has not let his disability stop him from embracing his loved ones, going to the footy and the races, and, unbelievably, standing up in front of audiences again. When he slowly makes his way to the stage he receives a standing ovation, and he deserves it. His body is not what it was, but his mind is as sharp as a razor. He also takes his message of hope and determination to the hospital bedsides of other stroke sufferers and, through his work for Men of League, to other footballers who are doing it tough.

John Peard was an inspiration to a generation of fans as a rugby league player, and even more today, as a stroke survivor, he is an inspiration. And not just to those battling illness, but to everyone blessed enough to know him.

When I visited John in Sutherland Hospital soon after he suffered his stroke, he looked up at me and said, echoing his words of thirty-four years before when we were young Roosters together, 'Don't you worry, Jack. I'll make it.'

And, once again, he has.

Fine thanks mate

Fighting Back

When I was just starting out in first grade, for Easts, in 1966, I had an interesting encounter with St George's peerless lock forward, John 'Chook' Raper. He was a treat to watch. Apart from his wonderful cover defence, Chook used the ball very cleverly. He'd do a little bit of shuffling and dummying around the back of the ruck or on the edges, putting guys through gaps or breaking away himself. In defence against Saints that day, I decided to position myself just off the ruck so I could read Raper's attack and try to shut him down. Chook took exception to my spotting tactics and after I'd tackled him a few times he got me a good one. He hit me high and down I went. As I lay on the turf he looked down at me and said, 'Get up, son, you're going to cop worse than that in first grade.' I struggled to my feet and played the ball.

Chook was right about copping more punishment – I was on the receiving end of plenty of biff over the years. But bruising physical encounters are part and parcel of rugby league. It's central to the game's allure, after all, and so long as it's not overly dirty, we thrive on it.

But nothing I encountered on the footy field prepared me for what happened to me in the first week of June 2002. I had a stroke and nearly died. I was paralysed down one side of my body, and spent many months in hospital. It took all my determination to fight back, but, like when Johnny Raper laid me low, fight back I did.

CHAPTER 1

Life and Near-Death

Crash-tackled

At age fifty-seven, I needed a kick in the backside, but I didn't need one as big as the kick I got!

Back in 2002, my life was just drifting along. A typical day for me would be a 6 am start on the road driving my concrete truck, delivering and picking up loads at building sites and concrete plants all over Sydney, chatting to people about footy or the races, telling a few jokes. It was a good business, owning my own truck, being master of my day. It wasn't heavy work, although I'd pitch in with a wheelbarrow on the site at the drop of a hat. The hard bits came when doing your runs on schedule as the traffic in Sydney got more congested each year, and the streets I'd known for so long all seemed to change. Suddenly a street that had been two-way for as long as I'd been driving it would be one-way and I'd have to detour. Or I'd hit a speed bump that wasn't there the day before.

Then, after knock-off time, around 4, I'd race down to my home away from home, North Cronulla Lifesaving Surf Club, and have a quick workout, lifting some heavy weights. I've always tried to stay fit, and as well as giving my cardio a boost with swimming and running, I'd really got into power lifting. After a few stubbies, I'd go to the pub or a club, meet some friends for five or six beers, then go home – my marriage to my childhood sweetheart Christine had broken up, though she was still my best mate – and cook my meal, almost always steak or fish and vegetables. (My dad swore by that tucker and he lived well into his nineties.) Then a bit of TV and off to bed so I could do it all again tomorrow.

I was too comfy in my existence. Growing old complacently. All my life I'd set goals, and as my seventh decade loomed I found myself without one, except to keep doing what I was doing. If anything, while in the past I'd channelled my energy into achieving at surf events, rugby league, setting up businesses and being an in-demand public speaker and raconteur, now I was putting my heart and soul into lifting weights.

I have some wonderful friends I've met through rugby league, and one of the greatest is a bloke named Bobby McMillan, who used to play half for Souths. Bobby and I both drove concrete trucks and would put in some time at the gym at North Cronulla, cool down with some beers, then hit the weights. We'd whack 150 pounds (68 kilos) on the bench-press barbell and compete to see who could do the most repetitions. As I'd been my whole life, I was so bloody competitive. Just like when I was playing for the Roosters or the Eels or Australia, or even doing laps on the training paddock, I *had* to win. Bobby would think he'd have me with twenty-nine reps and I'd pull off thirty. Which is a fair bit of weight, 150 pounds lifted thirty times. Our blood pressure was up because of the lifting, and alcohol was coursing through our bodies. We must have been bloody mad. Doing extreme lifting after filling yourself up with booze is like lighting a match over a tank of petrol.

Unlike a lot of former sportsmen who get fat and out of condition when their playing days end, I'd always remained trim and fit. It was a point of honour with me that I took care of myself and looked good. I had always been strong for my size. On the footy field, blokes would try to run over the top of me, thinking, 'Oh, he's only a little fella', and it gave me great satisfaction when I combined strength and good tackling technique to smash them.

Of course, in the end I got smashed myself, good and proper. I didn't see my stroke coming. I'd been invited by BHP to go up to Brisbane, all expenses paid, for three days and nights of big club and pub functions for the 2002 opening State of Origin match; the other guests were league greats John Raper, Reg Gasnier and Graeme Langlands. I felt good within myself, and eager to get into it. I'd be speaking and telling jokes at the events, interviewing Chook, Gaz and Changa, catching up with old mates, and partying hard. For me, a dream. I couldn't wait to get on that plane and pop the top on my first tinnie.

The three days went as expected. I consumed enough alcohol to fill Sydney's Warragamba Dam. My jokes and stories went down well, and the game, as is usually the case with State of Origin, was a cracker.

I didn't want the party to end. On the flight home, Reg, Graeme, John and I had more to drink. When we landed at Sydney, they caught cabs home. Not me. I'd planned ahead. I'd parked my ute at the long-term car park at the airport so I could drive straight to North Cronulla surf club for a workout and some weight-lifting. What the hell was I thinking? I should have gone straight home and slept off my big week away. But I was telling myself, 'Don't take the easy way, John. You've had your fun and games, now it's time to balance the ledger at the gym.'

At the club, I got straight into it. I picked up the 40-pound (18-kilo) dumbbells. One in each hand, doing clean and press with them – I know who was the bloody dumbbell! It was a tough workout and I was blowing like a southerly when I finished. Suddenly it seemed that the whole gym was spinning. 'Bloody hell, what's going on? This is a bit strange …'

There's a noticeboard on the wall there, listing the rules of the gym. I glanced at it but instead of the words I knew so well, all I could read was gobbledygook. And the sign was flashing in and out of silhouette.

I was unsettled, and very unsteady on my feet. I felt dizzy and a little nauseous. But did I take myself to the hospital? To a doctor? Did I go home to bed? I did not. Mr Bulletproof decided that what was happening to me was just an aberration, maybe a delayed hangover from Brisbane, perhaps a bug I picked up on the plane. I showered, got dressed, dropped my suitcase at my unit in Cronulla, and drove to the Businessman's Club in Caringbah, known as 'Bizzo's', where I'd arranged to meet up for some beers with my good mate Peter Cruikshank.

While there at the club, I put on a bet for myself, and for Changa and Chook, who'd given me a hundred bucks each before we said goodbye at the airport. The horse we backed was Through, trained by Kevin Robinson.

'How was Brisbane?' Peter asked.

I told him all the tales and then just mentioned that I was feeling a bit off. 'Peter, there's something wrong with me. I'm seeing stars and stumbling around.'

'Well, here's a plan: see if you can stumble your way over to the bar, because it's your shout!'

'But I'm seeing three things when there should only be one,' I told him.

'I bet when you order your beers there won't be three!'

Demolition Derby

Later on I drove home to Cronulla, went to bed and went straight to sleep. Sometime during the night, I had a stroke.

Next morning, Friday 7 June, I awoke and tried to get out of bed. I fell straight to the floor with a crash. What the hell was happening to me?

I decided that nothing was. Nothing *could* happen to me. I was fit and healthy and capable of drinking most blokes under the table and throwing around 150-pound dumbbells. In other words, I was in deepest denial. I had to get dressed and go to work. That's all there was to it. This problem I was experiencing, whatever it was, would soon pass. Bring on the day.

I attempted to put on my tracksuit pants but I couldn't lift my leg in. I fell again. There on the bedroom floor, I was writhing around frantically struggling to get my clothes on. It must have looked hilarious, but there was nothing funny going on this day. Finally I got my duds on. I dragged myself to my feet somehow, then saw my keys on the ground. I reached for them and down I went again.

Some minutes later, and by now unable to walk, I literally commando-crawled out of my front door and got behind the wheel of my ute. I had to get to work and pick up my truck. It's a measure of what was happening to my mind and my body that I kept going and didn't call for help.

I had no idea what a stroke was. Like most people, I thought it was some kind of heart attack or central nervous system condition, perhaps leading to paralysis. Cocooned in our wellness, we never stop to think much about illness. I never did, anyway. I thought I was invulnerable; nothing was ever going to happen to me. I would live till the age of 110, doing exactly what I was doing – working hard, lifting weights, drinking, yet always enjoying perfect health. For this reason, I simply didn't comprehend that I was having a massive stroke – what the doctors call a 'brain attack'. That I was on the verge of death.

I only learned later that a dissection in the carotid artery in my neck had stopped the flow of oxygenated blood to the right side of my brain, starving it of oxygen and damaging it terribly, and paralysing the left-hand side of my body. My left leg, my left arm, everything on that side of my body in fact, stopped working. I couldn't see out of my left eye, which is why, as I drove the seven kilometres to work at Taren Point, lurching all over the road, I collided with two signposts. Then, two kilometres from the garage at work, I smashed into the back of a parked cement truck. Its metal tray sheared the roof off my ute like a knife lops the top off a boiled egg, and missed my head by centimetres. Had it hit me, it would have taken my head clean off. I reversed, disentangling my vehicle from the truck, and … continued on. Nothing – my inability to use the left-hand side of my body or see through my left eye, the nearly fatal collision with the truck, the fact that my ute now had no roof – had registered.

It was a miracle that I arrived at my destination alive. I should have died on that deadly journey and it's an even more sobering thought that I could have taken many innocent people with me. When the car came to a halt I slumped forward onto my horn. Workmates came running and opened the driver's side door of my wrecked ute, and I tumbled out onto the ground.

I heard one bloke say, 'He's having a stroke', and, still in denial that anything was wrong, I insisted, 'No, I'm not.'

They carried me to the drivers' room and laid me on the lounge while someone rang 000. Thank God, Sutherland Hospital was not far away, and the ambulance was there within five minutes. I was admitted, and there I remained for the next four-and-a-half months.

When I was stretchered into intensive care, contorted, immobile and white, the doctors set immediately to work. Seems odd, but I could speak. If it's the right-hand side of your brain that's attacked, the power of speech is not affected. Problem was, in my dazed state, I kept calling the poor bloke in the bed next to mine Reg Gasnier.

My family was contacted, and the news they received was about as bad as you'd ever want to hear concerning a loved one. I wasn't expected to survive.

Funny thing, though – people told me later that when I occasionally regained my senses that terrible day, and they asked me how I was doing, I always told them the same thing. 'Fine thanks mate.'

I wasn't ready to drop off my perch just yet. I'd had a great life filled with love, humour and sporting achievement. And what inspired me to fight the most formidable opponent I'd ever faced were my hopes for the future and memories of the past ...

CHAPTER 2

Fortunate Son

My Early Years ... All Jokes Aside

Doing my stand-up comedy routine, I get laughs whenever I tell the audience that when I was growing up in Atherton, Queensland, my mum and dad were so poor that the woman next door had to give birth to my sister. I add:

We were so broke that we used to go to the KFC in Cairns and lick the other customers' fingers.

My parents were in the iron and steel business – she used to iron and he used to steal.

Dad was no rocket scientist. One day he pulled me aside and said, 'John, there are three kinds of people in this world. Those who can count and those who can't.'

I learned to swim at an early age. I had to. My six sisters and I slept in the same bed and they were bed-wetters. Mum would ask if I wanted to sleep at the top or the bottom end of the bed and I'd say, 'Mum, just throw me in the shallow end.' I'd wake up and there'd be a rainbow in the room.

To put food on the table, Dad had to get a part-time job as a Bible salesman. He was enthusiastic and hardworking, but he had one major drawback: a terrible stutter. It was typical of Dad that he turned his disability into a positive. He'd knock on someone's front door and when the householder appeared, Dad would say, 'W-w-w-would y-y-y-you l-l-l-like to b-b-b-buy a B-B-B-Bible or w-w-w-would you r-r-r-rather I-I-I r-r-r-read one t-t-t-to y-y-y-you?'

Ah, good old Dad. When I die, I'd like to go the way he did, peacefully in his sleep. Not like the three screaming passengers in his car.

Well, thankfully, life was nothing like that.

Once a Cane Toad

My father, who was also named John but known as Jack, lived to the age of ninety-seven and passed away only recently in a nursing home. I vividly remember him beach-fishing with his rod down at Bondi. He was a good fisherman, and his catches fed our family well. I swear he could catch a fish in the middle of summer with 3000 people swimming in front of him. He'd cast way out over their heads and he'd pull in a flathead, a bream, a whiting. He fished off the beach and the rocks until well into his eighties.

Our family was Dad, Mum, me, my sisters Margaret and Di, and my little brother Geoff, who came along nine years after I was born in tropical Atherton (that bit was true) in far north Queensland on January 15, 1945. Dad was stationed in the army there after World War II. Serving with 1 Australian Corps of Signals he'd done his duty in New Guinea, Egypt, Greece, Lebanon, Syria, Morotai and the Coral Sea. Even though wives and girlfriends were forbidden from visiting their men at the Atherton base, Dad, the ultimate wheeler-dealer, found a way to get together with Mum after he'd wangled her a job in the local post office. Nine months after Mum's arrival in Atherton, I was born. My sister Margaret has a letter that Dad typed right after I was born. It reads: 'Valda's just had our first child and he's wonderful!'

When Dad was demobbed we headed to Sydney to live with his mother in the western suburb of Auburn. That was where Dad and Mum had met before the war. Dad was a good pool and snooker player, and after a night mis-spending his youth in a local snooker parlour he staggered past a dance hall, looked under the door, saw a great pair of legs and decided to introduce himself to their owner. It was Valda Scott, my mum to be. 'Till the day he died he swore that Mum had the best legs he'd ever seen. (And he should know, having once won a lovely-legs competition himself). Dad went into the dance hall and asked this beautiful girl to trip the light fantastic. They fell in love.

Dad, Mum, Margaret, Di and I lived with my grandmother for five years in Auburn in a little house with chooks and a horse in the backyard (people were always yelling, 'Horse loose! Horse loose!') before we moved to Cammeray, on Sydney's lower north shore.

My Dad, the Antipodean Arfur Daley

We were a typical working-class family but still managed to have holidays at Woy Woy or Easts Beach, down the south coast near Kiama. That was a treat worth waiting for. Dad would go rabbiting with his pet ferret. He was an antipodean Arfur Daley. He'd tell us how when he was young he'd collect old newspapers and sell them to shopkeepers as wrapping paper for tuppence a bundle.

Dad was a gambler. His mother warned our mum, 'Val, do you know Jack gambles on the horses?' Over the years, his habit caused a lot of grief in our family. We'd probably have been a lot better off financially if Dad hadn't been a gambler. Whether it's hereditary or all my own doing, I don't know, but in spite of Dad's bad example I like a flutter too. My brother Geoff, as well. Sister Di plays the pokies. Margaret, the cerebral one in our family, takes on the stock market.

Dad was in his thirties when war broke out, and so was older than most of the soldiers. They called him 'Pop'. He sailed away on board the *Queen Mary*. His mother paid for a man in a boat to chug out beside Dad's ship as far as the Heads, holding a sign saying, 'Goodbye Jack!' but Dad never saw it because he was already below decks organising the crown-and-anchor game. He reckons he won big that day and right through the war, though I've got my doubts. He was also always a great collector but I don't think he ever collected anything that was worth much. Among his treasures were a bus ticket from Tripoli and a train pass from some other exotic place – of nothing but sentimental value.

He had a favourite yarn about his war days. It concerned the Colchester Cup, a big race that the soldiers held in 1941 in Palestine. About a thousand Aussies and Brits came from camps all around Gaza for a big sports day which included a wrestling tournament, running races and the Colchester Cup, a donkey race along a 150-metre track. The twelve donkeys were rounded up from the local sandhills and auctioned off, and the successful bidder got to ride. A bloke named Ted Weston bought one, but now had second thoughts about riding him. Dad, who'd dragged himself away from the two-up game he ran around the corner from a brothel, piped up, 'I'll ride the bugger.' There was no saddle or bridle so he'd have no alternative but to grab the donkey's neck and hang on for dear for life as his steed ambled along the 150 metres.

Just before the start, he sought a little local knowledge about how to ride a donkey. A friendly Arab told him that no matter what else he did, he shouldn't beat the animal, just nudge it gently. Off they went, the other riders whacking the tripe out of their braying mounts. Not Dad; he sat astride his mount, gently nudging it with a stick to keep it going in the right direction. As the other donkeys veered off-course and tried to bite their jockeys, Dad's sauntered across the finish line six lengths ahead of the nag that ran second.

Typically, he didn't win a penny. His donkey paid nine Palestine quid for the win but in Dad's pre-race excitement he had forgotten to put a bet on. He had to settle for the cheers of his unit and for getting well and truly tanked out there in the desert that famous afternoon. There's a photo of Dad taken with a box Brownie right after he won the Colchester Cup: a cheeky-looking bloke with curly hair sitting on his bored-looking donkey and holding his riding stick above his head in triumph.

Dad was a survivor. He could make the best of any situation. Even in the nursing home at the end of his life he worked the system to ensure he had the best time a 97-year-old ailing man with one leg possibly could.

Rugby League Wins My Heart

My lifelong love affair with sport began after we moved to Cammeray and I'd take myself off to North Sydney Oval on weekends to watch the matches there. Rugby union was played at the oval on Saturday and I'd watch men like Wallaby forward, lord mayor-to-be and future knight of the realm Nick Shehadie play. Then on Sunday I'd roll up again to sit under that big fig tree and watch the North Sydney Bears rugby league team. I enjoyed union, but league won my heart. My main man for the Bears was Peter Diversi, a champion hard-tackling lock who represented Australia. When the final bell sounded I would tear onto the field and walk proudly off with the players.

I can close my eyes today and suddenly I'm back in the 1950s cheering on the red-and-blacks. I would model my defence on Diversi's. He always wore number 49 on his back and liked to pick blokes up and drive them hard into the ground. Today I'm remembered for my kicking more than anything else, but I still consider that tackling was the strongest part of my game. At the annual Kangaroos dinner last year I went up and introduced myself to my childhood hero, who's still going strong. Here's to those mighty Bears of my youth – Kenny Irvine the flying winger who died way too young, Lenny Diett, Norm Strong, Peter O'Brien, Jimmy Gillon at halfback …

There were marvellous teams back then. Norths; the premiership-winning Souths sides captained by big Jack Rayner and with the flying Ian Moir on the wing; I loved Newtown, too. And at that impressionable age I saw the beginnings of the record-breaking run of premiership wins by St George – eleven between 1956 and 1966 – with the all-time greats Gasnier, Raper, Clay, Provan and Kearney. Being a young fan in that golden era, how could rugby league not have got into a bloke's blood?

The first football jumper I ever owned was a navy-and-white Shore private-school rugby union jersey. A lot of people probably thought, 'They've got money, those Peards. He's going to Shore, that kid.' In truth, Dad bought it cheap after seeing it in a bargain basket at Mick Simmons sports store. Me, I wore it because I loved it.

Backyard Warriors

When I was eight we moved across the Harbour Bridge to Dover Road, Rose Bay, not far from Bondi Beach. I played football barefoot after school with my mates in our big backyard, and in nearby Lyne Park and Barracluff Park. I still reckon backyard footy matches produce the best players. I think of the Johns boys, the Gidleys, the Walters kids, Alfie Langer and his brothers, all of whom grew up to be champions. We all mastered the fundamentals of attack as little kids. We learned to kick with both feet, we learned to handle well and, most importantly, we learned to tackle. Those games were no place for the faint-hearted: it was full-on. The intensity was greater than some senior matches I played in as an adult.

How I loved to tackle. As a kid and all through my senior career I prided myself on my defence. I always hoped that the biggest player on the opposing side would get the ball and run at me – I'd clean him up with a nice hard, low tackle. My technique was good. Sometimes I'd chase the bloke with the ball and he'd see me coming after him and just sit down on the grass. He knew I had every intention of creaming him.

The worst part of those pick-up matches was that they came to an end. When it got dark our mothers would be out calling for us to come in for dinner, after which Mum would say, 'Get straight into the tub. Look at your filthy knees, and those grass burns!' We hated to be called home and would have happily played on until midnight. I'm sure that's why Australia does so well in sport against England, where it's dark at 3 pm and freezing for half the year and kids don't get the opportunity to have fun outside in the sun or fresh air after school.

My Rose Bay Gang

My gang included Peter Moscatt, who grew up to be a first-grade hooker with the Roosters, mayor of Waverley, a Labor politician and union leader. When Peter and I were both in Easts' lower grades, the club held a ball. I asked Pete who he was taking and he told me he didn't have a date. I said, 'Then why not ask my sister, Margaret?' He took my advice and today he's my brother-in-law.

All we Peard kids attended Rose Bay Primary School (Margaret would become headmistress there in her final posting before she retired). As soon as that bell rang each day, I'd race to the park where all the kids would meet and we'd pick teams. There'd be Peter Moscatt and Bruce Francis, the future Australian opening batsman. Bruce wasn't much chop at rugby league, but by God he could play cricket.

In the long summer afternoons, we'd magically transform the grass strips outside our houses into the Sydney Cricket Ground. Among the kids making up the Australian and England teams would be yours truly, Bruce, and Doug and Peter Alexander, who played first-grade cricket for Waverley for years.

Today, of course, it's different. Life is more dangerous, more frenetically paced. Kids don't have the fun we had. We could roam the neighbourhood and ride our billycarts up and down Dover Road without fear of being assaulted or run down by some road-raging driver pissed off because he's thirty seconds late for an appointment. And big backyards, too, in the inner-Sydney suburbs are becoming things of the past as the old quarter-acre blocks, where you could hit a six or dash over for a try under the Hills Hoist, are being replaced by medium-density and high-density dwellings.

I was blessed to be one of those lucky kids who is naturally gifted at many sports. I wasn't too good academically, but I could play league and cricket, where I was a handy batsman. I was a good runner, with stamina. I won swimming races at Bondi Baths at the south end of the beach, near the Icebergs club, and in the surf. I could catch and throw as effortlessly as breathing. I loved sport. I admired the champions of the day and thought that if I trained hard and was very focused and dedicated, I could be like them one day. I guess the goal-setting that has driven my life and sporting career had begun even then. I believe that in this life you get what you go for.

A Small, Skinny Kid Takes on the World

My willingness to work hard at sport helped me do better than kids who were bigger and more gifted than I was. I was always the smallest kid by far in any team I played in. My lack of height and chronic skinniness drove me to show that I was as good as – no, better than – anyone else.

People were always making fun of my size. I left school in 1961 aged sixteen and Dad got me a job as a clerk at the Postmaster-General's Department in Martin Place. The blokes there were often having a go at me. 'Johnny,' they'd say, 'You can't work here. Child labour was outlawed last century!' That spurred me to show anyone who equated lack of size with lack of talent, skill and heart that I was as good as (and better than) bigger people. The laughter at first was the fuel for my dream to be a success at sport at the highest level – against the odds. It motivated me to try my best to be the best. I never slacked, always gave 100 per cent. To do otherwise would have been to cheat myself.

I was inspired to be a good footballer, too, by a teacher at Rose Bay Primary named Bill Goodman, who loved his league. I still see Bill around today. Rose Bay's colours were black and gold, the colours of the mighty Balmain Tigers. I was the tiniest lock and second row ever, but I insisted on playing in the forwards because that's where the action was and the tackling got done.

I met my lifelong friend Keiran Speed in the mid-'50s when we raced against each other after I'd joined Bondi Amateur Swimming Club at Bondi Baths. We would have been in primary school. I ran, swam and trained with Keiran around Bondi, Centennial Park and other parts of Sydney's east. We pushed each other to the limit and loved every moment of every day of our young lives.

In the block to the rear of my family's house in Dover Road was a public tennis court of red clay where they played competition tennis every Saturday afternoon and Wednesday night. Mum and Dad had a social hit there and I'd sit on the back shed watching the matches. The proprietor let me keep the court tidy (big of him, and he didn't pay me a cent). I was too small to push the roller but I swept the court and kept the sand off the sideline tape.

Back at the house, Dad painted a tennis net on the wall and I'd whack a ball against it with an old racquet. I enjoyed tennis, and it's a wonder I didn't take it up seriously. Another benefit of hitting that tennis ball against the wall was that it kept my eye in for cricket.

In my early teens I began lifting weights. It was unheard of for a boy to pump iron in those days. Not that they were state-of-the-art dumbbells. No, my weights were a pair of heavy old billycart wheels that I found in a garage somewhere. I attached the wheels to each end of an axle that I took off a fruit barrow. The weights were crude and rough, but they got the job done. I developed muscles where other kids had puppy fat, and I noticed in our footy games and wrestling matches that I was stronger than the other boys. I looked at myself in my parents' bedroom mirror and I liked what I saw.

After Rose Bay Primary, I went to Maroubra Bay High School (which, incidentally, got torn down for home units years ago). Our colours were Australia's green and gold. I played rugby league for my school during the week and for Kensington F grade in the Souths Junior League on Saturdays. I would have played seven days a week, twice a day, if it were possible. Lock was my position. That was ironic, because also playing for Kensington, in B grade, was Ron Coote, who went on to be one of the finest lock forwards the world has ever seen.

Swimming Training

All through my growing-up years I hauled myself out of bed to be at Bondi by 6 am for swimming training. If I ever slept in – and that was rare – Dad would be there to give me a kick-start. He'd come into my bedroom at 5.45, shaving cream all over his face, and bark, 'Righto, get up! If you leave now, you'll be there at six.' I'd pull on my swimming togs, whack a pair of footy shorts over the top, drape a towel around my neck, mount my pushbike and tear-arse through the backstreets of Rose Bay to Bondi, taking short cuts only local kids could know. There was no traffic then, so I'd make it in around eight minutes.

Waiting for me when I arrived was Keiran Speed and the swimming coach, an old bloke from Bondi surf club named Bill Douglas. Bill's strategy was not exactly complex; 'Away you go, up to the other end of the pool' was about the extent of it. But he was good. He instilled discipline in me by laying down the law: if you were late or didn't do your best at training you were letting down yourself and your mates in the surf club's R&R

(rescue and resuscitation) team. It was full-on, being in the Bondi Amateur Swimming Club team.

Swimming laps is bloody hard work, there were 400-yard (365-metre) time trials on Wednesday nights, and in the afternoon in the competition season we'd have marching drill on the sand. Can't say I enjoyed that much, but I did it because it was expected of me. If I had a choice I'd have been playing cricket or belting that tennis ball.

Bondi Days

For all the hard slog, Bondi Beach never lost its allure for me. My friends and I would be there having fun when we weren't training. When I wasn't able to cycle down, I'd run, or Dad would drive me. He was hopeless, though – always got the time confused – and on many occasions I was left standing on Bondi's Campbell Parade in the dark wondering where he was. Dad would drop us on Campbell Parade and then make arrangements to pick us up at a certain time. Between us we'd always get the arrangements mixed up. Dad would be waiting in his car at the corner and we'd be standing by the telephone box. Somehow, though, it was always the kids' fault and there'd be hell to pay.

Bondi Beach was our second home. Margaret, Di and I used to go to the beach at a much younger age than kids these days do. That's the sort of childhood we had. We were always at the beach. We could all body-surf and make monkeys of the waves on our surfer planes. We didn't have to unwrap our Christmas presents: we knew they'd be towels and cossies. Keiran and I would go board riding off Ben Buckler at the north end of

Bondi Beach. There are big waves out there, and surfboards didn't have leg-ropes in those days. So if we wiped out we'd have to swim all the way into shore to retrieve our boards, then paddle out again.

When I turned fifteen I was eligible to join a surf club, and, of course, Bondi has two: Bondi and North Bondi. The smaller blokes like Keiran and me, who were good swimmers, tended to join Bondi, while the bigger blokes signed on for North Bondi to be in its boat crews.

As a member of the surf club I was able to hang out in the recreation area, where they had weights and a shuttlecock court. Weight-lifting became an important part of my preparation for football and swimming, and even after I retired from elite sport in my mid-thirties, I kept pumping iron, until fate, in the form of my stroke, told me that I was bloody-well overdoing it.

I was very, very strong for my size. A bloke at the surf club named Charlie Gale, who was a former amateur wresting champion of Australia (and had ears so cauliflowered, people thought he was wearing a pair of tennis balls on the sides of his head), taught Keiran and me to wrestle. His lessons came in handy throughout my career when, at only eighty kilos wringing wet, I was constantly tangling with much bigger men. Charlie taught me to use leverage against my opponent so that the other bloke would end up on the bottom when he tackled me. He taught me how to fall so I wouldn't hurt myself, and how to use timing and momentum to smash a heavier bloke charging at me with the ball.

Keiran was every bit as dedicated as me to make it as a top sportsman one day. He called me 'Dissa', as in 'Dissa-Peard', and I nicknamed him 'Have-a-Chat' because he never shut up.

We were ultra-competitive with each other. We'd race each other on grass and in the water, and try to lift heavier weights. Keiran's dad, Ralph, had weights in his garage – a chin bar, a dip bar, dumbbells – and I spent a lot of time round at their joint in Ormond Street, near the Astra Hotel, pumping iron with Keiran and his brother Dennis, who died of a kidney ailment a few years back. Mrs Speed made us health shakes with eggs, peanut butter, malt and goat's milk. I don't know if they made us healthier, but they were delicious.

About Dad

People often ask me where I got the ability to stand up in front of a packed house and tell jokes or make motivational speeches. Blame Dad. He was into amateur theatricals. I have a photo of him wearing a black-and-white check stage suit. He loved the Tivoli Theatre, and went there to see the vaudeville shows in his lunch breaks when he was working in the city. He had a talent for making up little rhymes and that was his party trick.

There was always laughter in our house. Whether it was Dad pulling his schemes and stunts that somehow never worked out the way he planned, or the comedians we listened to on the radio and watched on TV, we learned the truth of the old adage that humour is the best medicine. Dad would double up at the antics of the Marx Brothers, the Three Stooges and Laurel and Hardy. Jimmy Durante was one of his favourite comedians, and we played a song by 'the Great Schnozzle' at Dad's funeral. He also loved the singing of Al Jolson.

He'd tell stories and people would hang on every word because he told them so well. People say I'm the same. I could always tell a yarn and cut a bloke up with a bagging, in a friendly sort of way.

My father was a rogue but also a bit hapless – which is a dangerous combination. He was always putting his head in his hands and moaning, 'Oh, I've ballsed it up again, haven't I?'

At Easts Beach caravan park, it'd take Dad hours to put up the annexe to our caravan. It was always falling on his head. Other blokes got their annexe up in minutes. One afternoon, Dad said to Margaret and me, 'Come down the beach, we'll do a bit of fishing.' When we got to the water we saw a group of local fishermen pulling in a big long fishing net, alive with fish. About a dozen holiday-makers were giving them a hand to haul the net in, so we three took a corner too and started pulling it up onto the sand. Every so often Dad surreptitiously plunged his hand into the churning mass of flathead, snapper and bream, grabbed one and stuffed it down his pants or in my and Margaret's T-shirt. When he'd pinched eight or nine this way, he whispered to me, 'Take the bloody fish and throw them into the long grass outside our caravan. But whatever you do, don't let the fishermen see you!' I did what I was told.

Finally when the net was ashore and the fishermen's catch was stowed in buckets, the head fisherman turned to all the holiday-makers and said, 'OK, you visitors to Easts Beach, thanks very much for your help today. We couldn't have pulled the net in without you. Now, to show our appreciation we'd like you all to help yourself to some fish for tea. Go ahead, take as many as you like.'

Then he turned to Dad and said, with a steely glare, 'Everyone except you! You've been stealing 'em and giving 'em to your young bloke all afternoon.'

Dad always thought he was pulling the wool over people's eyes, but usually the only person he fooled was himself.

Watching Giants Do Battle

One of my childhood treats was whenever Dad took me to the rugby league match of the day at the Sydney Cricket Ground, to see the Saints, the Tigers, the Jets, the Rabbitohs or my beloved Bears do battle. The great international matches, too. As a kid I saw the magnificent Great Britain and French teams of the 1950s and '60s. I was there, peeking through the picket fence, the day skirmishing broke out all over the field in the 1954 Great Britain vs New South Wales game and referee Aub Oxford abandoned the game. 'Jeez,' I thought, 'I'd like to get out there one day.'

I'd stand right down in front of the M.A. Noble Stand living in hope that the ball would get booted over the fence to me. Then, at the end of the game, once the players had showered, I'd be waiting outside the dressing room to gather autographs. After the last game of the year I'd ask the players for their socks as souvenirs. One, St George's Bryan Orrock, actually gave me his. In the early '70s, I asked the great English halfback Tommy Bishop for his socks after he'd played a match for Cronulla, to which he replied, 'What on earth would you want a Pommy's socks for?' I told him I'd collected them since I was a kid, so he handed them over. (Running home I dropped one and it smashed!)

I used to admire the wonderful English forwards of the '50s and '60s, in the days when they usually gave us a belting. The Poms and the touring French teams would always stay at the

Olympic Hotel at Moore Park, where the players would wash their jerseys and hang them over their windowsill to dry. Les Hayes, my friend and future Bondi United and Roosters teammate, and I would be hanging around down on the street; then, when the wet jerseys came out, we'd scale the side of the building and try to souvenir them. Les got a few, too. He was a tough little bloke and could really blue. Rather have a fight than a feed. Although, the jury's still out on how he would have fared if terrifying Great Britain players like Brian McTigue or Brian Edgar had been able to get their hands on him.

The Moose's Revenge

Since my stroke in 2002, my short-term memory is not great, but my long-term memory is excellent – better, if anything, than before. Memories of days at the footy fifty years ago remain in my mind as clearly as if they'd happened yesterday, and so do my recollections of those giants who played rugby league in the 1950s. For Easts, Bobby Landers, 'Straw' Andrew (whose career was ended with injury one big Newtown forward dropped him on his head), Bobby McDonagh, Bill Rooney, Doug Ricketson, Bruce Rainier, Billy McNamara, Dick See, Bob Heffernan and Terry Fearnley; for Wests, Jack Gibson, Keith Holman and Noel Kelly; for Newtown, Gordon 'Punchy' Clifford, Greg Ellis and Bobby Whitton; for Manly, Jack Sinclair, Roy Bull, who's passed on now, Billy Delamere, who also had a very bad stroke, and the inimitable Rex Mossop, who's still as strong as a moose.

I recall Rex, in his maroon jumper with the big white seagull emblazoned on the front, leaping high to take the opposition's kick-offs. He was a character long before he became a household name on TV. Once at Sydney Sports Ground (now Aussie Stadium), Rex was playing for Manly against the Roosters. It was a rainy day. At half-time he was trudging back into the dressing room for some oranges and, no doubt, a puff on his pipe, and there was a man in the crowd really giving it to him: 'You're a bloody mongrel, Mossop! You're the dirtiest player in the game! Go back to Brookvale Oval!' and other witticisms. Rex didn't break stride. He reached over to the bloke, calmly and precisely took the umbrella out of the man's hands, snapped it across his knee and handed the pieces back to his tormentor. That was the classiest thing I'd ever seen.

How Dad Kept Us Laughing

Yet if Dad had had his way, he'd have given the footy a miss and packed the whole family into our rotten old car and driven us out west to Blacktown or somewhere near there. He'd pull up by a paddock, get a stack of hessian bags out of the boot, and we'd all have to roam through the cow paddocks picking up cow manure and lumping it into the bags so he could spread it on his beloved garden at home. (Dad wasn't much of a gardener, but he enjoyed pottering around out the back with his flowers and chooks.) On our way home to Rose Bay, Mum, Margaret, Di and I had to sit on our evil-smelling cargo. It was a very small car and there was a lot of cow shit.

Once, when Wirth's Circus came to town, and after, someone had told him that elephant manure was very good for petunias.

Dad sneaked under the rope to collect some, literally from under the feet of the tethered elephants. The droppings were steaming as he spiked them and plopped them into his sack. Suddenly an angry voice rang out: 'Hey, mate! What the bloody hell are you doing? Leave those bloody elephants alone!' It was the elephant keeper. Dad ran for his life.

He kept us laughing every minute. I like to think I've inherited his mischievousness and sense of humour. When Mum died, far too young, a bunch of Dad's old army mates came to the wake in a little house in Bondi. They said, 'Jeez, you've got no idea how funny he was in the war.'

Jack Peard was also a punter and on Saturdays he worked for an SP bookie named Bruce up at Kings Cross. Mum never saw one penny of the money Dad was paid because he'd bet it all away as soon as he earned it. The bookie was raided by the police on a regular basis. There were blokes working phones everywhere on his premises. Dad told me that it was the way of the world that the bookie, the bloke who ran the show, got rich and the underlings, like him, were doomed to stay poor. 'Bruce comes to work in a Mercedes-Benz,' he said sadly. 'I catch the bus.'

Dad was very much the patriarch and when we sat up at the table for dinner we kept silent if we didn't agree with whatever he was saying. Dad had very set roles for husband and wife. He never cooked and he never let Mum wash the dishes. He welcomed the money that Mum was able to bring into the house, but in an old-fashioned way I believe he resented the fact that he wasn't the sole breadwinner. One Christmas, Mum bought Dad an electric mower. He was furious with her for spending the money.

About Mum

My parents were like chalk and cheese. As well as being beautiful (check out the photos in this book if you don't believe me!), loving and a superb cook, Mum was extremely intelligent. My father was a great family man in many ways but he was selfish too, probably a product of his generation in that he insisted on making all the family decisions without much consultation. When Mum, after working in a newsagency and a cement yard, got a job in a hardware store and she very quickly ended up being company secretary there, there was friction between them. Did Dad feel threatened by her success? Probably.

Yet they loved each other deeply. When they went to a dance, Dad wanted his best friends to dance with Mum because he thought she was so wonderful she would brighten up anyone's evening. He wanted to share his treasure.

Mum was the first person in Australia to computerise the inventory of a hardware store, and when you think about the number of different-sized screws and nails and things you'll understand what an accomplishment that was for a person without computer training or experience.

She was also very nurturing and one of my fondest memories of her is when we were all at Rose Bay. We had a laundry outside the back door and a copper to wash the clothes in, and there was Mum with the copper stick, wearing my shoulder pads under her dressing gown to soften them up for me before I played football for Bondi United. And in those days they weren't the light vinyl shoulder pads they have today; they were heavy leather ones, and stiff as hell until you ran them in. She was a small woman, but she looked huge with those pads on. She must have scared plenty of door-to-door salesmen.

Another time I had some new, light football boots made for me by a wonderful bootmaker in Crown Street, East Sydney, named Bill Connolly. Mum wore them around the house for days to soften them up for her precious boy.

I don't think it helped that, being so intelligent, Mum had to contain all her feelings, thoughts and emotions in our house. She never got angry with any of us, although she had plenty of reasons to. She bottled it all up. That can't be good for your health. I believe it contributed to her getting ill.

Mum died of leukaemia in 1988. She was only sixty-nine. Aside from the illness that killed her, there was not a thing wrong with her. She was very fit and swam every morning at Bondi while Dad fished.

Golden Child

My parents supported me to the hilt. No sacrifice was too much. They went to all my football and cricket matches and surf events. I was their golden child. In those days the first-born boy in any family was considered special, but my sporting prowess in spite of my diminutive size made me even more special in my parents' all-forgiving eyes.

When I was trying out for the 6 stone 7 pounds (41 kilos) Sydney City team at Redfern Oval, Dad stood right behind the selectors commenting loudly, in a bid to influence them to pick me, 'Wow, look at that kid! What's his name? He can play! I don't think I've ever seen a better schoolboy footballer!' Another time, when the linesman didn't turn up, Dad offered to run the line. When I went to kick a goal I swear his flag was in the air before my boot even made contact with the ball. The ref chipped him: 'Look, I know he's your son, but that *wasn't* a goal.'

We didn't have much money and most of whatever money that was spent on the children was, I'm a bit embarrassed to admit, spent on me. Mum and Dad truly believed that I would achieve great things in sport. My sister Margaret reckons I got a rails run in the family. That's true. I was trained to swim by the great Harry Nightingale at Bondi. Mum and Dad could only afford one bike, and of course I got it. I ate steak for dinner and my siblings were served chops or sausages. I liked Streets ice cream so everyone had to have Streets when they preferred Peters. Ours was a three-bedroom house. Mum and Dad had one bedroom, Di and Margaret shared, and until my brother Geoff made his appearance in 1954, I had my own.

Sadly, I cocooned myself from my family, selfishly obsessed with my dreams of sporting triumphs. When I paid my siblings attention it was usually to tease and torment. Margaret still ribs me about how I'd call her 'goggle eyes' because she wore spectacles, and how I'd throw them into dark places and laugh when she couldn't find them.

I rarely did anything around the house, while Di, Margaret and later Geoff had to pull their weight and mine as well. They all had to go to my sports prize-giving nights but I can't recall ever attending any of theirs. Such was the pecking order that I don't think they'd have expected me to go. And nobody ever questioned or resented the special treatment I received. It was just the way it was.

I was so focused on my sport that I'm afraid I wasn't terribly connected to the rest of the family. I tended to go my own way and live in my own world, playing little home movies in my head of holding a trophy high while being hoisted off some sporting field by my adoring team-mates. Geoff was a bit of a natural sportsman too, but unlike me he was one of those guys who was just king of the kids, never tried to be, just was. He was a born leader without ever trying to dominate in any way. People deferred to Geoffrey whereas I, being small, had to fight for everything I achieved. And that, I believe, is why I played for Australia while Geoff, who was a fine player and taller than me, never did.

I backed myself into an emotional corner with my family and it took ages for me to let my guard down and show them the love I really did feel but was unable to display. Even when I got engaged to Christine, whom they'd never met, they read about it in the newspaper. I was totally guarded and self-contained. Margaret tells me that when her husband Peter returned from end-of-season trips with the Roosters he'd update her with yarns about my hilarious antics; how I told a hundred jokes a minute and walked around with glasses without lenses, a big cigar and a baseball cap turned backwards. She was hearing about a totally different character from the one she thought she knew and she would say, 'Peter, no way. You must be talking about someone else. My secretive, serious brother has never told a joke in his life.'

My aloofness continued, I'm sorry to say, until 2002 when I had my stroke and, of course, my sisters and brother and their families put their lives on hold and made financial sacrifices to shower me with love and care, and I responded as best as I could. It took something so terrible to give me the courage to open my heart to them. Di remarked, when I was at my lowest ebb and unable to care for myself, that finally she felt she had her brother back.

Margaret assures me today that while I got most of Mum's and Dad's attention, she, Di and Geoff led happy lives. Mum went to the girls' school fetes and always spent far more than she could afford on their clothes. In time Margaret immersed herself in the academic life and went to university and then became a teacher. She lived at home until she was twenty-four, and married Peter Moscatt. Di, in her quiet way, was a rebel. She went out with boys earlier than Margaret did and got into the surfie culture. She ended up marrying Robert Conneeley, a junior world surfing champion whom she'd adored from the time they were at school together. Now they live in Margaret River, Western Australia.

Geoff lives in Wollongong these days and runs a disposal store. I told him, 'I need one of those camouflage jackets, Geoff.' He said: 'I got thirty-six of them in yesterday and I can't find one of them today.'

CHAPTER 3

The Boys of Summer

A Larrikin at Large

The greatest legacy my parents ever gave me was to bring me up in Bondi. In those days no one had cars, so you'd spend your whole day down at the beach, surfing, playing games in the clubhouse, forging friendships and creating mayhem. Once Bondi is in your blood it's there for life.

I was at the beach all summer long, and winter too. Keiran and I and our friends would have a surf in the morning no matter how cold, hang around the surf club, then, if it was a Saturday, catch a bus to the Sydney Cricket Ground for the match of the day. It was always packed on the Paddo hill, where we liked to stand, so we'd each take a couple of beer cans, embed them in the ground and stand on them so we could see over the sea of heads. After the game we'd get back on the bus and go straight to the Rex pub in Bondi for a beer and a spirited discussion of the afternoon's game. You could tell the blokes who'd been because they carried their programs folded up in the back pocket of their jeans as a badge of honour.

Until my stroke I surfed there whenever I could, even though in later life I lived twenty kilometres away. Keiran Speed to this day is down there for a surf at 5 am every morning, summer and winter, sunshine or rain. He'll be there at the crack of dawn until the day he dies. Keiran says his day goes downhill from the moment he finishes his morning surf.

I was a larrikin growing up on the beaches and footy fields and in the parks of the eastern suburbs, which was much more working class then than it is today. Nowadays even a small, ramshackle house is worth a million. There were girls and beer and parties, of course, but the priority for me was working hard to one day realise my sporting ambitions. I trained every day, every single day, to make sure I was the fittest bloke around.

Keiran and I swam countless laps in the baths and caught wave after wave from out the back right into the sand. We were fast, strong swimmers with impeccable and powerful strokes. We always performed a complete set of stomach strengthening exercises before we hit the water. We were always placed among the winners in races. Who knows, if we hadn't focused on football perhaps we could have been excellent swimmers.

Bondi junior R&R teams had a tremendous record of success thanks mainly to one man: Harry Nightingale. He was the swimming coach and he was terrific. We called him 'Salty'. His skin was deep brown, the colour of the outback desert, from being in the sun all the time, and the salt would dry bright white on him, which was how he got his nickname. He taught me a lot about swimming style, the best way to stroke and kick, and he was a precise drillmaster. He demanded nothing short of the very best.

Keiran and I were selected in the junior R&R team coached by Nightingale. In 1963 I was captain of that team when we won the Australian R&R Titles at Warrnambool in Victoria. The event was televised and my sister Margaret can remember the commentator saying, 'Oh, the tiny guy's won …' Winning the Australian championships was a very big deal then, as it is today. Not that being captain gave me anything special to do other than keep a little bit of discipline around the place and make sure we all got to training on time. At the surf club they called me 'the Mighty Atom'.

Aub Laidlaw, the Bondi Antichrist

There was always a bit of animosity between the surf club guys and the board riders, who saw themselves as outlaws and laughed at the red-and-orange costumes and caps and the regimentation of the clubbies. The surfies also hated the beach inspectors, who were always hassling them and confiscating their boards if they didn't have a registration sticker or when they strayed out of their restricted zone.

Aub Laidlaw, the legendary Bondi chief beach inspector who became infamous for measuring bikinis to ensure they didn't defy his idea of decency, was a strict and very tough old bugger. He was the Antichrist to the board riders. He waited for a surfboard rider to wipe out and lose his board – as mentioned, there were no leg-ropes in those days – and then he or his lackeys would race into the water and grab the board and lock it in the clubhouse until the surfie forked out a hefty fine. Lose your board three times in a day and you'd have to take a second job to pay your penalties.

One night someone went to the Bondi promenade with a can of paint, and next morning when Aub hit the beach he saw emblazoned on the path in huge red letters: 'AUB LAIDLAW IS A DRAG QUEEN'.

I didn't mind Aub, though I took care not to get on his bad side. I've always had a soft spot for hard but fair authority figures. Jack Gibson springs to mind, and Kerry Packer. Blokes who don't care if they're loved or hated but single-mindedly get the job done, whatever it takes.

Training to Win

Mick Souter, who was Jack Gibson's trainer at Easts when I played there in the 1960s and who later followed Jack to Parramatta, was an important guy at Bondi surf club. I swam against him, and Mick could swim. He was a huge, strong man, and he had a mate named Graham Elliott who was even bigger, and he could swim, too. I felt a little intimidated when my team had to swim out into the surf in the belt races and Mick and Graham and their guys would be in the alley next to us. They'd always get an explosive start in the race because they could run across the sandbank – the height difference meant that the water would only be up to their knees while it would be lapping at my waist and I'd have to push through it. So by the time we started swimming they might have twenty metres on us. I kept going, however, and at the end there'd never be that much distance between us. I was so determined, and that made up for many things.

I would never give in. Nor would Keiran. I knew if I was able to come in ahead of Keiran at running or swimming I'd have a good chance of winning. When we were lifting weights, I'd do fifty-one reps and he'd go for fifty-two. Our wrestling matches at the club were fierce affairs and would have done justice to Brute Bernard and Killer Kowalski at Sydney Stadium, although, unlike Brute and Killer, Keiran and I were for real. Happily, our battles for supremacy never harmed our friendship.

Running together was the glue of our friendship. The sport became a fad in the '60s but John and I were running in the mid-'50s when we were just boys. I'd like a dollar for every kilometre we ran together over the years. Must be thousands and thousands. We'd meet in the early morning at the big tree in Centennial Park to race over a predetermined course. Future dual rugby union and rugby league international John Ballesty and future Roosters prop Jim Hall sometimes joined us. After the run there was no putting our feet up; it would be back to the gym for weights or down to the beach for a swim.

My passion for training made me a very fit young man. I was usually first home or at least right up there with the leaders in any run through my sporting career, right into my thirties when I was up against blokes fifteen years or more younger. Even when I occasionally broke my rule and had had a big night out, I would never pull out of a planned run. When that was the case, Keiran would know immediately I was a bit under the weather and, sensing weakness, zero in on me like a jackal. He'd put enormous pressure on me when we were running those hills and I was feeling a bit iffy, yelling at me to run faster. I responded, refusing to let him get the better of me. I was quicker than Keiran over shorter distances, but he could beat me, though not by much and by no means all the time, over five kilometres.

Often when we were in our mid-teens we ran with groups of older blokes, guys from the surf club or the Eastern Suburbs Roosters who ran at the beach and at parks around our area. Once Keiran and I ran alongside Doug Ricketson, a tough and resourceful Roosters centre and the father of future skipper and international Luke, and Easts' first-grade halfback, Bruce Rainier, who would coach me for a while at Bondi United. Fit as they were, Doug and Bruce couldn't keep up with Keiran and me, even though we were wearing old Dunlop Volleys tennis shoes, and more than once we left Dougie vomiting his guts up over the railing on the promenade at Bondi Beach.

Getting into the Swing of the '60s

Keiran's and my competitiveness wasn't confined to sport. Back in the old days when we were young and good-looking (well, Keiran was), we both chased members of the opposite sex. As teenagers we naturally began noticing girls, the beautiful ones with brown skin and long blonde, sun-bleached hair who are ubiquitous at every beach and surf club in the world. It was around 1962 or '63 when we became aware of girls and the weird and wonderful way they made us feel, sometimes even causing us to forget for a while about footy or swimming. There was no holding us back.

There were always dances at the surf club and local pubs, and I courted the Bondi belles while pounding out a mean version of the stomp to the live music of Little Pattie, the Atlantics, the Deltones and a hundred bands who tried to be like the Beach Boys.

Being blessed with the gift of the gab, it was my job, when Keiran and I spied a couple of likely lasses, to do the initial chatting up. He would bide his time until I'd broken the ice with some slick patter or a joke, then he'd saunter in and claim the prettiest one for himself. It was a case of me doing the hard yards and him scoring the try.

We did silly things. At the Garie Surf Carnival down the south coast they bunged the keg in the beer tent after the event, and the big lark was to drink as much as you could and then run flat chat to the top of the huge, steep sandhills. The object was to make it to the top without chundering. As far I can recall, no one ever did.

One of our great hangouts was the old Rex Hotel, in Beach Road, Bondi. We knew the resident band and their set-list of surfing songs by heart. We knew when they played a certain song that their set was nearing its end and we took it as a signal to hit the bar before the rush and buy four or five longnecks to drink on the way home.

Partying by night was a good counter to my relentless training during the day. We often rocked up to a block of units we called 'the Concrete Jungle' at the back of Tamarama Beach. Every Friday and Saturday night there'd be a major party there that would last all night. At the Jungle they played the music loud, and everyone left in a cacophony of shouts, whistles and car-horn blasts. My God, I pity the poor neighbours who lived within earshot of the Concrete Jungle – and that included everyone in a twenty-kilometre radius!

A Sportsman Goes to Work

To help Mum and Dad put food on the table and support us four kids I left school early, at fourteen, and worked as a clerk at the PMG by day and studied at tech at night to get my third-division rating, which would put me at the same level in the public service as a kid who had gone on to do his Leaving Certificate. My first pay packet was three pounds, six shillings and ninepence a fortnight.

Nowadays league is fully professional. Blokes are paid huge money to train every day and represent the club. In my era, we were paid peanuts and couldn't have survived, let alone provided for a family, without a day job. When I was eighteen, in 1963, I left the GPO and went to work for the Customs Department. Dad knew someone who worked there and he pulled a few strings and arranged an interview for me. I was employed as a customs clerk.

I was happy at my new job. I quickly joined the Customs Department's league team, which played in the very competitive public service comp in Sydney's Domain at lunchtimes. Our matches were pretty willing, especially when we played the Police Department, which had a lot of grade players in its ranks. We won the competition one year, and my great friend Peter Cruikshank was in the same team.

And, even better, in the Customs office I found myself sitting opposite the most beautiful girl I had ever seen. Christine Rivett was lusted after by half the blokes in Customs, but when I asked her out, she said yes. She lived at Hurstville, which is a long way from Rose Bay, especially if you don't have a car, which I didn't when we first dated. I racked up a lot of travel. We went to the pictures and to dances at the surf club. We went to the football and spread out a picnic blanket on the hill for our lunch. She turned up to see me play for Bondi United and later got on well with my Roosters team-mates' wives and girlfriends.

I was selfish, obsessed by succeeding in sport, and it couldn't have been easy going out with someone as focused as me, but Chris hung in there and in 1968 we were married.

CHAPTER 4

United

I Set My Sights on League

One night in 1963 a group of us from the surf club were down at the Rex Hotel and a fellow from Bondi United junior rugby league club was running around trying to recruit players for C grade – that's for blokes under eighteen. I said to Keiran and my other pals, Allen Dibben and Johnny Shirley, 'Let's all go and play for United.' There were enough of us clubbies to form a second Bondi United side in the C grade under-nineteen competition, and we'd be known as the C2s. The C1s wore green jerseys with a white V, and the C2s a white jersey with a green V. The comp had already started so we were right behind the eight ball, but we won match after match, and against all the odds we made the grand final – against our own C1s. They *just* beat us.

The next year the best players in the C2s were promoted to the C1s and we won the grand final against Paddington Colts. I was captain and five-eighth, and John 'Monkey' Mayes, who later played for the Roosters, Manly-Warringah and Australia, and remains a close friend, was our halfback.

Keiran and I could run kilometre after kilometre without becoming breathless, but neither of us was the fastest bloke in town, so to put on a bit of pace over a hundred metres (essential for rugby league), we hooked up with the veteran sprint trainer Jim O'Donnell, who was in our surf club. Jimmy trained the champion sprinter and rugby union and rugby league international Michael Cleary, the rugby international Alan Cardy, my mate Peter Cruikshank, and some other champion runners at the Reg Bartley Oval at Rushcutters Bay. Two nights a week Keiran and I would go down to the oval, by the Harbour and just down the hill from Kings Cross, and run sprints and 400s with Jim and Michael and the pentathlon team for the '64 Olympics. We couldn't keep up with these speed machines, but none of our footballing peers in the junior league was doing intensive training like this. Jim O'Donnell drove us hard, and Keiran and I, as usual, drove each other even harder.

Suddenly rugby league was the sole focus of my sporting ambitions. I put all my energy into this wonderful, brutal, unforgiving and rewarding game. There can't be a tougher sport on earth, with the possible exception of boxing, and anyone who plays league has my respect.

Bunny Reilly

We used to play down at Centennial Park a fair bit, against such teams as Clovelly, which also had a good number of surf club guys, and Paddington Colts, which had a good number of street thugs. Those games against the Paddo Colts were bloody hair-raising affairs.

The most fearsome Colt of all was a short, light lock who was as hard as nails and had the best tackling technique I'd ever seen. If he got his hands on you, he'd hurt you. This little bloke was a real intimidator, always in the thick of it when the fists were flying, as they invariably did when we played Paddington Colts. Before a game in the dressing sheds, as we pulled our jockstraps, boots and shoulder pads out of our airline bags, all our blokes would want to know the same thing: 'Is Bunny Reilly playing today?' If the answer was yes, gloom would fill the room. A belting was inevitable that afternoon.

Of course it was Barry 'Bunny' Reilly's mission to shut me down. As United skipper and five-eighth, I directed most of our team's attack. We had some wonderful battles and, as usually happens when two players go hard at each other, animosity turned to respect, which evolved into a lasting friendship. We were good mates when we both joined the Roosters and played in the same teams, and we're good mates today. Bunny came to my dad's funeral, which I really appreciated because it couldn't have been easy for him to get to the church. Bunny these days spends most of his time on his back with a serious kidney ailment and has to have dialysis twice a week.

Bondi United's All-Star Team

In 2005, to mark Bondi United's sixtieth anniversary, an All-Star Team was selected from all those players who'd worn the green and white down the decades. The team was as follows: at fullback, David Thompson; wingers Doug Ricketson and Wayne Miranda; centres Les Hayes and Ray Beavan; five-eighth Kevin Junee; halfback Johnny Mayes; lock, yours truly, John Peard; second-rowers Ferris Ashton and Luke Ricketson; props Paul Dunn and Bob McDonagh; and hooker Peter Moscatt. I'm proud to be in that company.

On the Road to Senior Football

After two years with Bondi United, Keiran switched codes and joined Eastern Suburbs rugby union, but I continued to train with him every day. Strangely enough, we would both go on to make our first-grade debut in the same week in July 1966, him for Easts rugby union and me for the Eastern Suburbs Roosters league team, and we each got picked out of position. I was a five-eighth and he was a centre but we both got stuck on the wing. We also both won premierships, me in 1974 and '75 and Keiran in 1969.

In 1964 and '65 I was selected from Bondi United to play for Easts' President's Cup team, a virtual rep side picked from all the junior league teams in the district. Of course Bunny Reilly and Johnny Mayes made it too, and for Monkey and me it was good to have Bunny on our side for a change.

We always used to draw Souths in the President's Cup and, with such future Rabbitoh greats as Bob McCarthy, Arthur Branighan, Paul Sait and Eric Simms, they had the strongest junior league of all. There were always will-o'-the-wisp Aboriginal kids in their teams. These guys were incredibly fast and so skilled.

Once in a curtain-raiser at the Sydney Cricket Ground we scored under the posts against the more fancied Souths and shot to a 3–0 lead. I was the goal kicker and lined up the simple conversion attempt, fifteen metres out and right in front of the black dot on the crossbar. I dug a divot – no kicking cones in those days, not even a sand-boy – and placed the ball straight up. It was one of those slippery yellow leather footballs, not the easy-to-grip synthetic ones they play with today. I placed the ball, and took seven steps back. This, remember, was before around-the-corner kicking; you approached the ball straight on and kicked straight with the toe of your boot.

I moved in, connected sweetly … and missed the goal! Amazingly, both linesmen put their flags up, signifying that I'd kicked the two-pointer. I can only assume that each must have thought he was dreaming when the ball skewed sideways, surely no one could miss such an easy shot. The Rabbitohs fans went ballistic. I pointed to the scoreboard. It read 'Easts 5, Souths 0', so I *must* have converted. Of course, we didn't stay in the lead for long. Souths overhauled us and won 13–5.

Any time I played Souths I knew I was in for a pummelling. Those blokes in the red and green were tough and they were good, products of their district. Newtown and Balmain were the same, until they became extinct. It's sad to think that of the three, only Souths remain as a first grade-team.

Throughout 1965, Monkey Mayes, Bunny Reilly and I were called up into Easts' third-grade team when some of the regulars got injured. We'd been targeted as future first graders and the Roosters' selectors wanted to blood us to see if we could cut it in senior football. Third grade in those pre–salary cap days was often where first graders returned from injury and also a haven for former first-grade stars who were getting on in years. These old blokes may have been slower and heavier than in their heyday, but they'd lost none of their killer instinct and they delighted in crunching us young guys. It was a huge leap from President's Cup to grade and many a young star from junior league days found it too hard and gave the game away.

One of the very first games I played as an Easts lower grader was against Wests at Pratton Park. After my game was over I hung around the dressing room hoping to catch a glimpse of a man who had become, like Peter Diversi, a hero to me: the legendary Wests hard man Noel 'Ned' Kelly. Ned was one of the old school; a ferocious front-rower for Wests and Australia with a short right that ended any on-field argument quick smart. There wasn't a player in the game who wasn't wary when he shared the field with Kelly. He was at the end of his career that day, but his scary aura, exacerbated by a weird patch of white hair at the front of his dark thatch, had not diminished. I wasn't game to approach him, but later we became friends. Ned clashed with all the other tough guys of the day, such as Saints' Billy Wilson and Kevin Ryan and Souths' John Sattler, but, as is the way of rugby league, he never failed to seek them out after the game for a beer to swap war stories and ensure there were no hard feelings – until next time.

Captain Blood

Ned's cohorts in that very strong Wests side included Nev Charlton, Billy Carson, Kevin Smythe, Mark Patch and the aptly named Dennis Meaney. They had a firebrand second-rower named Jim Cody. He was only twenty or so in the early '60s, but his youth didn't deter him from waging war on his opponents. Jim would punch, bite, kick – whatever it took. One of the all-time great rugby league yarns concerns Jim and Billy Wilson. It was the 1962 grand final, Wests vs St George. In the first half, Cody knocked Saints' great skipper, Norm 'Sticks' Provan unconscious. Sticks was carted off. Billy assumed the captaincy. At half-time of a very tight game, Billy addressed his men: 'Now listen, we all know that Cody got Norm, but I don't want anyone trying to get square. We're already a man down [there were no replacements in those days] and we can't afford to have anyone sent off. Now remember: no get squares! Anyone who gets himself sent off will have to deal with me.'

St George kicked off to start the second half. Cody chased the ball. Billy chased Cody. Bang! Cody was carted off, away with the pixies, and referee Jack Bradley gave Billy his marching orders. Seems that when he had the chance to avenge his team-mate, he couldn't resist. Saints won anyway. That's how good they were.

Here's another terrific, and true, 'Bluey' Wilson story. He broke his arm in another match against Wests but, not wanting his team to be a man down, he refused to go off. By the way he was catching and tackling one-armed, the Wests blokes figured that his arm was hurt and singled it out for punishment. At half-time, Bluey came up with a ploy. He wrapped his good arm in bandages so that Kelly and co. would attack it and leave his busted arm alone.

Billy was a great man and a formidable sight on the field. He ran with his shoulders back and wore the biggest shoulder pads you could get. His head was always bleeding, which led to his other nickname, 'Captain Blood'. Billy played on into his forties

– an incredible effort for a prop – and he died young, of a cerebral haemorrhage.

Regular Rooster

I wanted to play first grade so badly. As well as my work with Customs, I drove a truck to make ends meet and on its side mirrors I fastened stickers that read 'First Grade', to maintain my focus. Every time I checked the road behind me, my dream was reinforced. I kept a pair of running spikes tied to the bonnet and a stopwatch in the cabin and whenever I drove past Queens Park or the Waverley College running track I'd slip the spikes on and do four laps of the oval.

In late 1966, aged 21, I did become a regular first grader, though there were times when I regretted it. Even though we had two Kangaroos in the team, centre Ron Saddler and halfback Kevin Junee, and some handy players such as fullback Allan McKean, centres Peter Dickenson and Jimmy Matthews and five-eighth Gwyl Barnes, that was the year Easts' first-grade team failed to win a single match. We won the wooden spoon convincingly. The team that came second last, Norths, were fifteen points ahead of us on the premiership ladder.

This was the darkest season in the Roosters' otherwise proud history. Never before or since had the club failed to win at least one game. Funny thing was, though, we'd come last the year before but managed a couple of wins and consequently the leagues club was already struggling – no one comes back to celebrate a loss – so if we had won our share of games in 1966 the $120-a-man winning bonuses could have sent the club plummeting into the red.

I learned of my call-up from the lower grades to the firsts this way. One night at training the Roosters' first-grade coach, an Englishman named Bert Holcroft, who'd been a handy player in his day, came up to me and said, 'Peard, you're in first grade this Sunday. You'll be on the wing.' That was the good news. The bad news was that we'd be playing the mighty St George Dragons, who had won ten straight premierships. And worse, I'd be marking the great international winger John King.

I was so nervous I hardly slept for the rest of the week, and only picked at my food as I worried how I'd measure up on the weekend. When I told Mum I'd be playing on the wing she fretted, 'But John, don't you have to be fast to play in that position?' 'Yeah, Mum,' I said, 'or big.'

There wasn't much chance of me stacking on the kilos in just a couple of days, but I thought I could at least improve my speed. Maybe then King wouldn't make me look a complete goose. This was my big chance and I wasn't going to blow it. Jim O'Donnell wasn't available so I called Mike Agostini, who, when he was running for Trinidad, had made the final of the 100-yards sprint at the Melbourne Olympics in 1956. He had made his home in Australia and trained sprinters.

'Mike,' I said, 'it's Easts' new winger, John Peard, here. I'd love to join your running squad.'

'You want to get faster for next season, do you?' he asked.

'No,' I said, 'for this Sunday.'

'I'm a sprint trainer, mate, not a miracle worker!'

Come game day I took my position on our right wing. Opposite me, at the old Sydney Sports Ground, was John King, Australia's left winger and the second-leading try scorer in the comp. Marking him was a daunting prospect, but things could have been worse. Had I been picked on the left wing I would've been taking on Eddie Lumsden, Australia's right winger and the competition's *leading* try scorer.

As things turned out, I survived the experience. The ball didn't go King's way, though Eddie Lumsden scored two tries on the other flank. In fact I only had to tackle King once, and fortunately there was a forward on hand to help me out.

I only got a few touches of the ball myself, and had to go looking for it. In a break in play I whispered to our halfback, Kevin Junee, that the next scrum we won I'd race in from my wing and, instead of him passing to five-eighth Gwyl Barnes, he should slip the ball to me. Saints would surely be caught offguard and I'd split them right up the middle.

Sure enough, we won the scrum and Kevin passed me the ball. But Brian 'Poppa' Clay, Saints' bald pocket battleship of a five-eighth, was wise to me. He waited till I had the ball then he grabbed one of my legs. Their big forward Elton Rasmussen took hold of the other and they hoisted me up. I yelled to referee Col Pearce, 'Christ, what do I do now?'

'Sonny,' he said, 'make a wish!'

Saints' great lock forward John Raper was a master. Wonderful cover defence, and incisive in attack. Just playing on the same field as John and his team-mate the brilliant Reg Gasnier made me a better player.

'I'm Savin' Meself for Trainin"

What a year that was, 1966. Not only did we lose every game, but we lost by huge margins. You had to laugh, and some of my better jokes came out of the adversity we faced back in '66, when the only thing we won all year was the toss. First time we did, we ran a lap of honour.

We were a young, small team under coach, Bert Holcroft. Bert was a good bloke who'd coached in the bush a bit as I recall. But the team was on a losing streak. At training, Bert would blow his whistle and yell, 'OK boys, take up your usual positions!' We'd all retreat behind our try line.

Bert was a tough coach, as I remember. He would make us run laps after regular training to equal the number of points we'd been beaten by the previous weekend. Fortunately Bunny Reilly and I were still mainly reserve graders when Manly beat our first-grade team 53–0. The poor blokes who'd taken part in the massacre had to run 21.2 kilometres and it was damn near midnight when they finished circling Sydney Sports Ground. As it happened, a bunch of those fellows pulled out of the following week's match with sore muscles and shin splints and Bunny and I were promoted to take their place. We never looked back.

Understandably, the seemingly endless losing streak affected team morale. At half-time against Wests I looked over at our Pommy prop Tom Higham and he didn't have a speck of dirt on him. 'Tommy,' I said, 'not doing much tackling today, mate?'

He replied, 'No bloody way, laaad, I'm savin' meself for trainin'!'

A Sandwich Short of a Picnic

There's no kind way to say it, some of the blokes in our team were a sandwich short of a picnic. One evening one of our forwards confided to me over a beer that he was having a little trouble achieving an erection when he was in the sack with his wife. Ever helpful, I said to him, 'Mate, I've heard if you drink a bottle of stout every day, it puts lead in your pencil. Why don't you try it?'

He looked at me and replied, 'Peardy, I haven't got time to write to women!'

CHAPTER 5

Jack's Law

Enter Jack Gibson

After my promising end to 1966 when I became a first-grade regular, I couldn't wait for Jack Gibson to take over from Bert Holcroft as coach of the Roosters in 1967. I'd heard Jack was very special and I was hoping to blossom under his coaching. Sadly for me, I missed all of '67 after contracting glandular fever.

When I got sick I copped a double whammy. Not only was season 1967 lost to me, but I found myself broke. At the end of 1966 I'd taken three months' leave without pay from the Customs Department so I could train seven days a week and get super-fit for footy. Shortly into my leave, I was stricken with the glandular fever. I wasn't sacked from Customs but I couldn't work for many months. I languished in bed at home at Rose Bay for four months, sick, miserable and skinny. For an active bloke like me, this was like being in prison. Luckily, when I was well enough I was welcome at Roosters training and in the dressing sheds at games. During this time I got a close-up look at Jack Gibson, the man and his methods.

Jack was a cut above other coaches. What I saw him achieve at the Roosters in 1967 inspired me to make it in this bloke's rugby league team as soon as I was up and running again in season 1968.

Thomas Edison said that many of life's failures are people who did not realise how close they were to success when they gave up. Well, the much-lampooned Roosters of 1966 didn't give up. They hung in there, and were blessed by the arrival in 1967 of a good coach who, using pretty much the same cattle as the year before, took us to the four-team semi-finals, finishing fourth in the comp. We went from laughing stock to premiership contender in a single season.

When Jack Gibson played for Easts, Newtown, Wests and New South Wales, from 1953 to 1964, he was a hard-arse of the ilk of Noel Kelly and Billy Wilson. As a coach he was completely the opposite. He forbade illegal play, knowing it only hurt the team turning on the biff. Anyone throwing a punch or committing any kind of cheap shot in a Jack Gibson team was dropped, no questions asked. He wanted good citizens on and off the field.

He drummed into us that the ref was *always* right (even when he was wrong) and we weren't allowed to back-chat him or sledge an opponent. 'One thousand Philistines were slain by the jawbone of an ass,' he'd say, 'and two thousand football games have been lost by use of the same weapon!' He'd pull a back-chatter straight off the field. He preached bone-rattling but fair defence and mistake-free football. He demanded that we play for each other. He turned us around, just like that. He exemplified the declaration by Indira Ghandi, who was prime minister of India at the time: 'There is no magic – only hard work, an iron will, clear vision, and the strictest of disciplines.'

Jack often had a chuckle when questioned about his Jekyll and Hyde persona. 'Coaches coach what they couldn't do,' he'd say. 'I couldn't play the game clean, but my teams have to.'

Jack was never one of the boys, and we respected him for that. Respect has to be earned, he always said, and he earned ours through his wisdom and the standards he imposed. Some people feel they can demand respect and yell and scream, but they're wrong.

He could intimidate without saying a word. When he wanted you to come clean about something, he'd just grip you in a steely stare and wait. Blokes would babble out everything they knew.

Things I Learned from Jack

I loved it, I couldn't get enough discipline. Training started at 6 pm and Jack demanded that we be in our training gear and out on the field at that time, not still strapping on our boots or getting a rubdown in the dressing room. That all had to take place in our own time, not his.

Jack had this idea that rubdowns made players sleepy and too relaxed, so he banned them from our dressing room. Years later when he was coaching the Cronulla Sharks he arrived for his new club's training session on a Tuesday night and was dismayed to find the change rooms crammed with rubbing tables.

'What the hell are those things?' he asked.

An old trainer didn't catch Jack's vibe. 'Jack, they're for rubdowns. I massage the players before games.'

'Well, I don't want my blokes falling asleep on the field,' Jack said. 'Get rid of the tables – I don't want to see them here on Thursday.'

Luck, Jack used to say, is 'preparation meeting opportunity'.

Another thing I learned under his wing was to set goals. Not only immediate goals, but medium-term and long-term goals, and to let nothing stand in the way of achieving them. I set goals for football, hoping to play to my potential, win a grand final and represent Australia. And I applied them to life away from the game. I aimed to be one day happily married with kids, run a successful business, develop myself as a person, maybe not be so self-centred as I had been.

Jack was never one of those fire-and-brimstone coaches who make Churchillian speeches. He was forthright, to the point, and he kept his message simple: tackle, kick and chase, perform the basic fundamentals of the game correctly, and don't make mistakes or give away penalties. Years later when Michael O'Connor was picked on the wing for New South Wales in State of Origin, he asked coach Gibson what defence the team would be using that night: up and in, mark-up or slide? 'Son,' rumbled Jack, 'just tackle the bloke who's got the ball.'

I have a theory that coaches are more verbose these days because players generally are much younger and need to have things explained to them. In my era, the average first grader was around twenty-six to twenty-nine. I didn't even become a regular first grader until I was twenty-two, whereas nowadays if you haven't established yourself by the age of nineteen or twenty you probably never will. Today Arthur Beetson is a talent scout for the Roosters, and if I say to him, 'Hey Beetso, I've heard of a likely kid from Cowra – he's twenty-three', Arthur will reply, 'Forget it, too old.'

Gibbo the Mind-reader

Jack Gibson was as smart as a whip. At the beginning of season '67, just before I came down with the glandular fever that would end my season before it even started, he asked me which of our halfbacks I would prefer to play alongside: Kevin Junee, a speedy, mercurial player, or John Mayes, my old Bondi United mate, who was more of an organising and defensive halfback. I replied, 'Jack, they're both good friends of mine. I'd rather not answer your question. I'm happy to play with either.'

'Well, then,' continued the cunning bastard, 'which bloke would you *least* like to play against?'

'I'd hate to play against Monkey,' I answered. 'He'd belt me and nip at my heels all day long.'

'Thanks, Peardy,' Jack said with a grin. 'You've just answered my first question.'

Jack had studied the great gridiron coaches and made many a trip to see them in America, and he pinched a lot of his classic quotes from them. That was OK. Such American football truisms as 'When you haven't got the ball, defence is all you can do' and 'You don't worry about a bloke's size – you can win with big blokes, you can win with small blokes – so long as they can play' apply as much to rugby league as gridiron.

Small blokes. Gibbo always had good little men in his teams: Bunny Reilly, Kevin Stevens, Harry Eden ...

Discipline, Tackling and Statistics

To put it mildly, Jack was a revelation. He emphasised defence, smart football and playing for your team-mates. He also instilled discipline where it was needed.

I believe today that without discipline there can only be failure. Whether you're a sportsman, a creative person, in the armed forces, at school or in business, you can have all the natural talent in the world but if you're not disciplined you'll never realise your potential. I'd always been disciplined since the days when I'd drag myself out of bed at 5.30 to swim or run endlessly around Centennial Park with Keiran Speed. Pushing myself to achieve had begun as a means to an end and become a way of life for me. But Jack made me more disciplined still, and I have used his lessons all my life, as a coach, as a businessman, and as a stroke survivor. It's a hard call to describe Jack Gibson in a single word, but if I had to, that word would be 'disciplinarian'.

He was also smart enough to realise that rugby league is a simple game. Back then, four tackles and kick. So if you could hold on to the ball for three and then kick intelligently and chase hard and wait for the other team to make mistakes, you were usually home and hosed.

He also taught Easts to tackle. The huge scores other sides put on us in 1966 became a distant memory in 1967 and '68, Jack's first stint with the Roosters. It was nothing for us to repel wave after wave of attack in our own quarter.

He also believed in statistics. Tackle counts, unforced errors, metres gained each set, points for and against, facts about the opposition – the sheets denoting this vital information became Jack's Bible. And this long before any other coach. Jack was the great rugby league innovator of his time.

'Craven As at the Kiosk'

Players would have walked on blazing coals for Jack Gibson. His word was their command.

There was a handy lower grader knocking on the door of first grade during Jack's first reign at the Roosters. One night in a pre-season game against Wests at Lidcombe Oval he was sitting on the bench for first grade, hoping against hope that he'd get a run. Suddenly Jack called out, 'Hey you …' The bloke leapt to his feet and started stretching, sure he was about to make his first-grade debut.

'You, son,' Jack repeated. 'Craven As at the kiosk.'

The kid, though somewhat shattered, shot off to buy the smokes on the double because of his respect for Jack.

Happy Hooker

My brother Geoff was a very handy footballer. He played halfback in the lower grades at Easts, which, with me and our brother-in-law Peter Moscatt also Roosters, made for a very family affair. One day Peter was playing second grade against Canterbury-Bankstown at Belmore Oval in 1975 and broke his leg in the first minute of the game. A replacement hooker had to be found, and pronto. Jack Gibson cast his eye around the dressing room, where Geoff and the other under-23s Roosters were refreshing themselves with a beer after their game. 'Who can hook?' Jack demanded.

Geoff had hooked for Eastern Suburbs Bays under-nines so he stuck up his hand and said, 'Mr Gibson, I can hook.'

Jack barked, 'Well, get your shin pads on and get out there.'

First scrum he stuck his head in, Geoff gulped, 'Oh, Jesus!' The opposition front-rowers were the huge and rugged Phil Charlton and the bruising Kiwi international Bill Noonan. For good measure, former international Geoff Connell was glaring from the Bulldogs' second row at the rookie hooker.

Luckily for Geoff, Les Hayes, who was good enough with his fists to have been a pro fighter, was in the Roosters' scrum and just as Charlton, Noonan and Connell were about to get stuck into Geoff, Les said, 'The kid's a friend of mine, so lay off him. Now, boys, are we going to fight or play?' The Bulldogs wisely chose the latter option and Geoff lived to tell the tale.

Jack the Fixer

Jack had a colourful life outside football. He'd worked as a bouncer in some very tough establishments around Kings Cross and he had contacts everywhere. If you needed a car, Jack knew a bloke who would sell you a good one cheap. Not that you ever had the opportunity to specify the make, vintage or colour, or even to check it out before buying. Jack would say, 'Turn it up, Peardy. You want a good car, don't you? This bloke sells good second-hand cars. You don't need to inspect it. What are you gonna do for Christ's sake – kick the bloody tyres? Trust me. You want a car. My guy will get you one. Leave it to him.'

Sheer Genius

I wanted to interview Jack for this book, but unfortunately he's not well these days. So the next best thing was to have a chat to Ron Massey, who was Jack's right-hand man through his coaching career. Ron is one of the most astute rugby league men there is. When I asked him why Jack was able to turn the Roosters' fortunes so quickly and decisively after he arrived in 1967, Ron thought hard before replying.

'The reason Jack made a difference there,' he began, 'is that he had his own ideas on coaching. When he was a player he was a very rough and frequently dirty fella. He did everything exactly the opposite when he was coaching. He would not allow cheap shots, figuring that league was tough enough as it was. He didn't need hotheads who were going to get penalised and cost the team, and play contrary to what he had come to believe was the spirit of the game.

'Jack emphasised how important it was to do the simple things right, to get the defence in order, to take tackle counts of players so that he could tell whether they were putting in. At first a lot of rival coaches thought that Jack's techniques were a joke. They said, "Oh we don't believe in tackle counts and all that other nonsense he's always spouting." But a particular coach who just happened to be one of Jack's staunchest critics was interviewed in 1968 and asked why he dropped a player and he came straight out with, "Just have a look at his tackle count." So he'd obviously come on board with Jack's way of thinking even though he'd never have admitted it.

'Jack was very much a club man,' Ron continued. 'He believed in players who believed in their club rather than themselves. Therefore all of the players in the lower grades were treated the same as the stars in first grade. Whenever possible, the lower-grade players would train with the first graders, so they wouldn't feel out of place when they were promoted to the top grade. When Jack brought a player up to do a job, like when he promoted the unknown John Rheinberger to play centre in the 1975 grand final, he fitted into first grade seamlessly, and played just as well as the established stars.

'Being such a knowledgeable bloke, Jack knew who could perform when it mattered and who couldn't. Jack left Easts at the end of the 1968 season, and then Easts let you, John, and Bunny Reilly go to St George and to Cronulla respectively in 1972. But when Jack came back to coach the Roosters in '74, the year they won the premiership, he brought Bunny and you back with him. He knew what you could do. He knew that you were going to help him deliver that premiership.'

Billy Buckingham, Medico

Another of Jack's trusted confidants was the team doctor, Bill Buckingham. Jack listened hard to Bill before he picked the side, and often made replacements mid-match after a quiet chat to the doc. In one game a forward had taken a knock but seemed to have recovered, and in the dressing sheds at half-time Jack asked Bill if the player was fit enough to play the second half. Bill said to leave him off.

'But he looks OK to me,' the coach offered.

'Jack,' said Bill, 'have you seen his tackle count? He's doing fuck-all. Leave him off, he's having a bastard of a game.'

Old Billy Buckingham was one of a kind. He was an excellent jazz musician and a damned good medico. Afflicted by Bell's palsy, on game day – I suppose so he wouldn't frighten the players when he had to get up close and treat us – he would wind Cellophane around his head to hold up his sagging dial. Well and good, but did that mean he was stitching us up one-eyed? His ever-present cigarette belched acrid smoke in our face as he stitched and snipped.

If we'd been hurt in the weekend's game, we had to roll up on Monday mornings to his practice in Darlinghurst, to get a medical clearance. Some of us joked we left Billy's surgery in worse shape than when we arrived.

'I'd Vote for It'

The dressing room was the scene of some great Gibbo one-liners. After one match that we should have won but, due to silly mistakes on our part, including dropping the ball with the line wide open, we didn't, the journalist Ernie Christensen fronted Jack with his notepad and pen poised.

'Coach Gibson,' he said, 'what do you think of their execution?'

Jack replied, 'I'd vote for it.'

Break Curfew

One of Jack's unbreakable rules was that his players had to be out of licensed premises by 9.50 pm, ten minutes before closing time at most pubs, and we weren't to get drunk in public. One Tuesday night after training a bunch of us went to the Phoenix

Hotel in Woollahra. Soon our props Ian 'Boof' Baker and Kenny Jones started arguing, as props tend to do. The disagreement continued outside onto the footpath, where Boof and Kenny swung haymakers at each other. Monkey Mayes and I did our best to separate the combatants but without success. They were big, strong blokes and right into it. I said, 'Bloody hell, Monkey, what'll we do?'

'We've got to split,' he replied. 'It's 10 to 10 – Jack's curfew. We have to get out of here. We'll leave them to it.'

So we got into our cars and drove down to the Sutherland Shire, where we were both living at the time. In our haste to make tracks, we were pulled over and booked for speeding. The cop breathalysed us but we were under the limit. When I got home, I thought, 'Oh, shit. I'd better ring Jack and tell him what's happened. I don't want him to hear the story second-hand. The blue, getting booked for speeding ... he'll think we were all pissed and it will be twice as bad for us as it is now.' I made the call.

'Jack,' I said, 'John Peard here. Monkey and I got into a bit of strife tonight.'

'Like what?'

'Well,' I stammered, 'we got booked for speeding after training.'

'Did they breathalyse you?'

'Yeah, we were both OK.'

'Good. I'll see you Thursday night, six pm, ready to train. Oh, and one more thing,' said Jack. 'Who won the fight?'

I was flabbergasted. How could he possibly have known about the brawl? He must have had spies everywhere. All I could stammer before hanging up was: 'Well, Kenny was slightly ahead on points when Monkey and I left *at ten to ten*!'

Lessons for Life

There's no doubt in my mind that a lot of the atrocities committed today by players simply wouldn't happen if they had a disciplinarian like Jack as their coach. He demanded that his players behave themselves off the field as well as on it. Anyone who defied him would be cut loose. No getting drunk, no fighting, no making obscene mobile phone calls (not that they had mobile phones in the '60s), no dirty jeans and T-shirts and baseball caps. We had to be polite and well dressed in public. We had to wear a jacket and club tie whenever we appeared at a function or appeared at a shopping centre or radio station to accept an award. 'Give Grace Bros the respect they deserve,' he'd say. That lesson has stuck, too. When I speak in public these days, or do anything involved with rugby league, I wear a coat.

Jack used to say, 'An idle mind is the devil's workshop.' You only have to look at the headlines to know that players today are prone to getting into strife. We've had numerous recent scandals involving rugby league players binge-drinking and abusing women, not to mention the hijacking of a street-sweeping vehicle. Today's players have no job but plenty of money and lots of idle time to spend it in. They live for today and setting goals is not on their agenda. The fans and the clubs and their managers tell them they're gods and a lot of them believe it. After all, most of them are just kids with a wonderful talent to play football. They haven't had the setbacks and hard knocks that teach wisdom.

Frank

The Roosters' results and morale immediately improved. We played and trained hard, but enjoyed lots of good-fun socialising with each other as well, like at Jack's Red Faces talent quest nights, where attendance was compulsory. I would always do a comedy turn, sometimes sending up footy broadcaster Frank 'It's long enough, it's high enough' Hyde and race caller Ken 'London to a brick' Howard.

My impersonation of Frank (who, as I write this, is doing it very tough at the age of ninety with a stroke and cancer) was always a hit. I'd sit behind a jimmied-up microphone with '2SM' on the front, wearing a pair of heavy glasses, and I'd say, just as Frank used to all those years ago on his broadcasts: 'Those boys standing in front of me – sit down! I can't see a thing! Goodness gracious, don't the mothers of Redfern teach their children manners? Son, let go of that microphone cord!' Or: 'Oh, look at Balmain ... Words fail me. All their forwards are standing around in the backs! Get those forwards back into the pack!' I'd present a Seiko watch to my best and fairest player, and then sing 'Danny Boy'.

When I took off Ken Howard, I was always interrupting my phantom race call to present a word from the sponsor: 'At the first sign of a cough, sniffle or a hangover, take my tip – buy Arthur Beetson's APC, the perfect panacea. Speedy relief for anything that ails you.'

When they made Frank Hyde, the doyen of league callers, they threw away the mould. Both he and Ken, I am reliably informed, took my mimicry as a compliment. Which it was.

Fight Night

Bondi surf club staged regular boxing nights to raise money for the club and we Roosters were encouraged to strap on the gloves for a good cause. One surf club fight night sticks in my memory. Newtown and Manly's Allen Maddalena went the distance with Jack Barrows; Balmain forward Dave Cooper wrestled Roosters forward Greg Bandiera (it was a terrific tussle – both blokes were strong, fit and knew how to wrestle); and I was drawn to box a handy pug from Papua New Guinea named Paul. My 'manager' was Boof Baker.

Boof was a good bloke, but, jeez, he was a prankster. Just before my match, he went over to my opponent, Paul, and said, 'Listen, mate, this is just an exhibition match tonight. Your opponent couldn't knock the skin off a custard, so go easy on him – just spar around, maybe throw a couple of left jabs to make it look fair dinkum.' Then Boof came over to me and said, 'Jeez, Peardy, what did you do to Paul? He's really got it in for you. Your only hope is to beat him to the punch. Get in there and hit him on the jaw as hard as you can. Finish him before he finishes you.'

I did as I was told. My love tap, unfortunately, only served to give Paul the shits. He knocked me straight down.

'Half a Dozen Crownies, Mate'

We used to go away on a lot of end-of-season trips in those days. Our club boss, Ron Jones, was always wangling jaunts to exotic locations like Bangkok, Hayman Island or Hawaii. We went to Singapore six times, and stayed at the very plush

Shangri-La Hotel. I'm sure when players from other clubs were talent-scouted by our selectors they'd pipe up, 'Look, I don't want to play for the Roosters, but can I sign up for a trip to Bangkok?'

One day we were all in the pool at the Shangri-La and ordering beers. 'Half a dozen Crownies, mate,' we'd say. 'And make sure they're cold.' It was as hot as hell in Singapore but the beer was always warm.

Boof Baker was a terror on our trips away. He came up with a cute trick. He'd drink his beer, then fill the empty bottle up with pool water and bang the bottle-top on again. Next thing he'd call over the waiter and tell him his beer wasn't cold enough and to take it away and bring him a replacement bottle pronto, and to make sure it was cold this time. That way he got many beers for the price of one, and some poor tourist that night would order a beer with their green chicken curry and get a mouthful of pool water.

CHAPTER 6

This is the Big League

In 1968 I recovered from glandular fever and was champing at the bit to resume my footy career with the Roosters. Johnny Mayes and I trained hard in the off-season, pushing each other on, just as Keiran and I had done in past years. When I ran onto the field at five-eighth in the first game of the year I had never been fitter, both physically and mentally, and it paid off. I had probably my best year in '68, winning the JJ Brown Memorial Trophy for Easts' best first-grade player, and was selected to represent Sydney Seconds against Country.

In his gruff way, Jack took me under his wing. That was no secret. He liked the way I trained at one speed – flat out –

exhausting myself every session, and how I stuck to his no-frills game plan in matches, tackling everything that moved, especially chasing the ball when it was our kick-off. I was no superstar like Gasnier or Raper, but I was wholehearted. If Jack had confidence that you'd give him all you had to give, you'd make his team every time.

One of my first games was under lights on a Friday night against the premiers, Souths, at Redfern Oval. There I was, the big crowd baying for Rooster blood, waiting for the kick-off, facing such formidable Rabbitohs as John Sattler, John 'Lurch' O'Neill, Bob McCarthy, Ron Coote, Elwyn Walters, Bobby Moses, Bobby Grant, Denis Pittard, Eric Simms and Mike Cleary, and thinking, 'Shit! What am I doing here? This ain't Bondi United. This is the big league.'

As fate would have it, I had a good game and got a write-up in the Saturday paper. The blokes at the surf club took me up to the Astra on the hill at South Bondi and bought me a celebratory beer.

'If You Get Hit on the Jaw, Cop It'

The write-up, and my growing reputation, was a blessing and a curse. Suddenly as Easts' playmaker I found myself a marked man and had to be wary of high shots and king hits in back play. The problem was fuelled by Jack's edict that no one could retaliate in a way that would draw a penalty. Some clubs, like Souths, knew that and whaled into us with immunity. Other clubs had designated enforcers to protect the little guys. Not Easts. And Jack was immovable about dirty play and get squares. The way he figured it, it was tougher to cop a cheap shot and turn the other cheek than to do your block and start a brawl. Jack would say, 'If you get hit on the jaw, cop it.' And he'd add: 'Let the referee decide. Put the pressure on him. It's easier for him to send two blokes off than one.'

I have lost count of the times I was knocked out in 1968. I know my brother has a number of photos of me being carted off in Disneyland throughout the year. The caption of one reads: 'John Peard, Easts' star five-eighth, is carried from Sydney Sports Ground after being dumped and knocked unconscious in the 13th minute of the game against North Sydney on Sunday.'

Inevitably I learned to play smarter; to stay away from the marauders while still dictating play. Jack left me to work things out for myself. He didn't spend much time on the nitty gritty of each player's game. He was more into ensuring that the entire team played as a cohesive unit: tackling hard, playing mistake-free percentage footy, and minimising penalties and errors.

The Smartest Thing I Ever Did

Two good mates from the team were Kevin Ashley, a goal-kicking second-rower, and Kenny Owens, the hooker. Kenny was the publican at the Exchange Hotel in Oxford Street, Darlinghurst. We used to go there after training a fair bit – probably too much.

Once I told Kenny I'd like to buy a house and own a pub. It was a bit of a tradition for footballers to buy into hotels, for better or worse. Kenny told me, 'Don't worry about pubs or houses now. How the hell would you pay them off? Get yourself a concrete truck first. There's a lot of building going on in

Sydney, and if you work hard and you have luck, your business will buy you the pub, and a home as well.' Listening to my mentor, Kenny, was the smartest thing I ever did. And Jack Gibson, who always insisted his footballers be hard workers, approved. I got myself a truck and signed on with the Farley & Lewers company.

'Jeez, You're a Nasty Little Bastard'

Bunny Reilly was another good pal. We'd come a long way from our Bondi United–Paddington Colts rivalry. Jack Gibson became a lifelong fan of Bunny the day he took on Wests enforcer Noel Kelly. Ned was having the time of his life, doing what he always did – terrorising rival forwards, slipping passes, charging into the rucks with fists and boots flying. Then … wham! Bunny, in one of his earliest first-grade games had bided his time awaiting the opportunity to lay one of his specials on the big man. Suddenly everything was in alignment. Bunny flew through the air on Ned's blind side, caught him around the legs, lifted him up and dumped him hard. Ned spat the grass and dirt out of his mouth and gasped in bewilderment, 'Jeez, you're a nasty little bastard! Where the hell did you come from?' Soon Bunny was known as 'the Axe', for reasons obvious to anyone who witnessed, or experienced, his tackles.

'Larpa' Stewart

We had a very special winger in those Easts sides of the mid-to-late '60s. His name was Bruce 'Larpa' Stewart, and he was an Aboriginal flyer, the original Black Flash, whose speed and twinkling footwork brought him a cartload of tries and made him one of the game's real personality players. Larpa could have played representative football had it not been his misfortune to play in an era of great wingers such as Lumsden, King and Wests' Peter Dimond.

Larpa was a jack-in-the-box off the field as well as on it. At the start of season 1968 I'd had Bill Connolly, the bootmaker from Crown Street, fashion me a new pair of super-lightweight boots. I believed that they would help me to run faster. They didn't, but boy, were they comfortable. These boots were so light and soft you could actually screw them up into a small ball that would fit in the palm of your hand. Anyway, in the dressing sheds after a pre-season game against Souths at Redfern, played in 35-degree heat, I took my new boots off and discovered that the intense heat and my sweat had made the black dye run. My feet were pitch-black. I scrubbed and scrubbed with a wire brush but couldn't shift that dye. Larpa Stewart strolled over and said quietly, 'Peardy, I tried that twenty years ago and it didn't work.'

High Praise

In 1967 and '68 Easts were an efficient little outfit. A good, small side. We didn't drop the ball. We chased on every kick. Our defence was the best in the league. We frustrated other more-fancied teams because we kept plugging away and wouldn't lie down. They ran on thinking, 'We should be able to get over this mob.' But they just couldn't. I was pretty typical: no superstar but a good all-round player who could set up plays, kick a bit, tackle and chase. I was faster than most people gave me credit for. And I played at 10 stone 12 pounds (69 kilos). We made the semis both years, and it was a four-team series then, so qualifying wasn't easy. Both times we fell at the penultimate hurdle.

I thank Jack Gibson for putting me on the football map. When Saints knocked us out in the 1968 semi-final, Jack came out in *The Sun-Herald* and said, 'Peard, he's the best footballer I've ever seen.' I don't know why he said that, because we both know I'm not. But I cherished the rap, and wish I'd kept the clipping to frame.

Man of the Moment

I have, however, kept another clipping, from the now-defunct daily newspaper *The Sun*. In an article titled 'The Man of the Moment: How Midget John Peard Became a Giant', league writer Peter Muscatt wrote:

> A Sydney youngster who once had a complex about his stunted growth, now strides the Australian rugby league scene like a giant. The spectacular rise to fame this season of Easts' 22-year-old five-eighth discovery, John Peard, already reads like a Grimm's fairy tale. Seven years ago, Peard was a midget of 4ft 11in and 5st 10lb wringing wet, hardly the credentials for a successful career in football.
>
> Peard had already left school and workmates chided him about his size and urged him to become a jockey. 'I suppose they were pretty close to the mark,' Peard recalls. 'I must have been just about the smallest bloke in the world for my age. If I wasn't going to become a jockey it looked like I would have to join a circus.'

Suddenly Mother Nature smiled on Johnny Peard and he started to grow. Inside three years he had nearly doubled his weight and grew to the thoroughly adequate height of 5ft 8in. 'I was just late in developing and I was very relieved when I started to gain those pounds and inches,' he said. Now he could make it in football if he was good enough.

At 18 he was in Easts' President's Cup team, and the following year was appointed captain before being called up to play the last six games for the club's third-grade side. The next year, 1966, when Easts first went through the horrors of losing every game, Peard started off as third-grade captain and graduated through the reserves to play the last three matches with Easts' top team.

Then came another setback as illness threatened to end his career in its infancy. Peard suffered a bad case of glandular fever and was bedridden for four months. He was then allowed to return to work but his doctor warned him he could do nothing strenuous for at least twelve months and his future in football again looked bleak.

In November last year, his doctor finally gave him the all-clear to resume light exercise and Peard started on the hard road back, firstly with long walks, then with jogging and finally with a course of weight training. He soon regained the three stone he had lost during his illness and after exhaustive trials, Easts' officials were finally convinced Peard was completely recovered and capable of resuming his grade career.

Since the start of this season, Peard has rocketed to stardom and after consolidating his place as Easts' regular first grade five-eighth, won his way into the combined City

Seconds team. That blooding in representative company worked wonders for Peard's confidence and his form since has been exceptional. There is no denying that had Australia's 19-man World Cup squad been picked now instead of a few months ago, Peard's name would have been among the chosen few. He proved last Saturday that he has now progressed beyond the stature of an outstanding prospect by more than holding his own with Australia's World Cup five-eighth, Bob Fulton of Manly.

The outstanding feature of Peard's game is his rock-like defence, but he is no slouch in attack either, and has developed a brilliant combination with Easts' Kangaroo halfback, Kevin Junee. Easts' officials, aware of Peard's football talents, recently signed him to a new contract for three years after this season. Peard's sporting activities have not always been restricted to football, as he was once a star surfer and at seventeen was a member of Bondi's junior R&R team which won the national title at Warrnambool, Victoria. Now working as a customs clerk, Peard is going steady with a girl he plans to marry 'in the near future.'

'No Daughter of Mine Is Going to Marry a Footballer'

I'd been seeing Christine for over five years by the time we were married, at St Andrew's Church at Hurstville in December 1968. Typically, I neglected to tell my family that we were engaged. They had to read about it in the newspaper. I meant no insult. After going out together for a few years, Chris and I just decided to tie the knot and it all happened so quickly. I thought, 'Why muck around? If I hold off much longer, someone else will get her.' Thank goodness Mum, Dad, Margaret, Di and Geoff turned up. It was mainly a family affair, Christine's and mine, with a sprinkling of sporting friends such as Keiran, John Mayes, Kevin Ashley and Kenny Owens. At the reception, the speeches were funny and the drink flowed.

There's a story I like to tell when I do my comedy act today. It's not true, but it should be. I say that when I asked Christine's father, Reg, for her hand in marriage he was outraged. 'Over my dead body,' he said.

'Why?' I plaintively asked.

'Because no daughter of mine is going to marry a footballer!'

I asked him to reconsider but he was adamant. 'OK, then,' I said, 'but, Reg, you've never seen me play. At least take this complimentary ticket for Sunday's game against the Rabbitohs at the Sydney Cricket Ground.' He took the ticket and came to the match, which we lost 48–0 after Denis Pittard cut me to pieces.

Afterwards, Christine's dad turned up in our dressing room. 'John,' he said, shaking my hand, 'I've reconsidered. You have my blessing to marry Chris.'

I was dumbfounded. 'Why have you changed your mind?' I spluttered.

'Because I watched you play today, and you're no footballer!'

Christine and I honeymooned on South Molle Island. It was an idyllic time, swimming, snorkelling and playing tennis with the woman I would be spending the rest of my life with. Funny how things don't work out the way we plan.

Our first home was a little brick house at Mortdale, deep in the St George district. It was opposite the footy field where the famous Renown United junior team played. Renown was the club of Saints stars of the 1950s and '60s Reg Gasnier, Billy Smith and Johnny Riley. I spent a lot of time perfecting my kicking in that park. Later, Christine and I moved to President Avenue, Kogarah, then Blakehurst and finally Cronulla. I made a living driving my concrete truck around Botany.

Our daughter Johanna was born in 1971 and Amanda came along four years later. I was a doting Dad. I was so excited after Chris gave birth to Jo in the Women's Hospital in Paddington that I turned up at the front desk next morning with flowers and said to the receptionist, 'My daughter gave birth to a wife last night!'

A New Coach for the Roosters

Jack Gibson had only signed on to coach the Roosters for two years, and we had a new coach in 1969, Louis Neumann. Louis was one of that now long-gone breed, the player-coach. He was a South African who'd most recently played for Leeds in England. Louis was the grumpiest coach I'd ever met. He would bellow at us, 'You, come here!' A ball-playing prop and second-rower, Louis would scream at us to run off his passes. A few blokes did, and you should see their heads today. No one threw a hospital pass like Louis. He was a tough bugger.

Louis was an uncomplicated coach, totally untroubled by tactics or tackle sheets. Discipline was not really important. He encouraged each player to run his own race. The house that Jack built was demolished in no time. Even though we had Saddler and Junee, Bill Mullins, Mark Harris, Jim Porter, Allan McKean and John Walker in our side, we didn't make the semis in '69.

A Match to Remember

Neumann lasted only a year as coach, but continued with us as a player when Don Furner took over in 1970. That year we only missed the semis by a point. By that time Arthur Beetson had joined us from Balmain, and Donnie Furner, who was very knowledgeable, was instrumental in getting Artie fit and me chosen in the Sydney Colts team (even though I was twenty-four!) to play the excellent Great Britain touring side, the last Pommy outfit to win the Ashes.

One of the most remarkable games of rugby league ever played took place in season 1970. When Easts lined up against St George at the Sydney Cricket Ground on Monday, 15 June, the Queen's Birthday holiday, the new four-tackle rule was being taken to task by fans and the media for having spawned haphazard, helter-skelter play with none of the strategy, control and planned moves of unlimited-tackle footy. It was a crunch game for us. We weren't travelling too well, in fifth place, and Saints were coming second, behind Manly. We were rank outsiders to win, but we proved our detractors wrong. We turned on nine wonderfully executed tries (Billy Mullins got three) in a 37–23 victory, and St George were no slouches either, crossing for five beauties. Play swept from one end of the field to the other, and the crowd was entranced. Those who saw that game still consider it one of the finest exhibitions of attacking rugby league ever turned on. Suddenly limited-tackle football didn't seem so bad.

Artie's and my great days were down the track but it was good to have him at the Roosters. I'd played against him for a few years and had enormous respect for his skills and rugged attitude. Of course, any animosity ended at full-time. You find most football players are friendly with each other. There's such respect for blokes who play our tough game. That's the beauty of football.

A Few Broken Jaws

Not that there was any love on show the day we played Manly at the Sydney Cricket Ground and Louis Neumann, John Quayle – who would go on to be one of the code's greatest administrators – and yours truly were sent off in a nasty clash. I was marched for belting Manly lock Billy Bradstreet. It happened this way: I kicked ahead and chased and Bill did what he was legally entitled to do, turn his back and keep me from the ball. I was frustrated because we were losing the game and I whacked him in the ear. Referee Keith Page blew his whistle and screamed, 'Off!' Mayhem ensued. I'd no sooner arrived in our dressing room when 'Canon' Quayle, a squeaky-clean player who'd never been sent off in his life, walked in, closely followed by Louis.

I adhere to the rugby league code that, generally speaking, what happens on the field should stay on the field, and a beer and handshake after the game should bring an end to hostilities. It's always intrigued me that the very rugged John Sattler was so outspoken against John 'Sleepy' Bucknell, who punched him and broke his jaw in the Souths vs Manly grand final in 1970, when Satts whacked more opposition players than I've had breakfasts. Manly's Malcolm Reilly was the same. Ron Turner kneed the fine English lock in the hip and wiped him out of the 1973 grand final against Cronulla. But Mal had earlier that year smashed Ron's jaw, just as he dented the skulls of Bob McCarthy and

Easts' own Bill Mullins, father of Russell, who missed a Kangaroo tour when he shattered the right side of his jaw in a collision with Reilly. Mullins attempted to get square and rushed at the Englishman. Result: Billy broke his left jaw. Arthur Beetson often tells of the time Manly were playing Souths and Paul Sait and George Piggins decided to gang up on Reilly. They waited till he ran the ball up, then tore in on him, fists clenched and cocked, from opposite sides of the ruck. Without breaking stride, Reilly waited till they were upon him, then lifted both his elbows simultaneously and belted them both on the jaw. Bang! Bang! Down went Paul and Georgie.

I played against Mal and Satts many times, but kept out of their way. Mal could mix aggression with skill, being a beautiful passer and kicker of the ball. It's unfashionable to say so, and Jack Gibson would disagree, but enforcers like Sattler, Reilly, Noel and Peter Kelly, Arthur Beetson, Les Boyd, Les Davidson, Mark Geyer, Steve Roach, Gorden Tallis, Carl Webb, Mark O'Meley and Adrian Morley add colour and drama to our game. They're good to have around, as long as you're not on the receiving end!

Time for a Change

My season in 1971 was ruined by a serious knee injury. It was my last for the Roosters – for the time being. Easts snared Australia's Test five-eighth Phil Hawthorne from St George, which left me without a possie. I'd moved to the St George area, I was in awe of the Dragons' feats, and I was mates with a number of their players, so when they asked me to join them to replace Phil, I accepted.

The old team was breaking up. Monkey Mayes left for Manly-Warringah, taking his place, alongside Bob Fulton, Mal Reilly, John O'Neill, Graham Eadie, Max Krilich and Ian Martin, in a terrific team that would soon win the comp. And my old friend, the Axe, Bunny Reilly, joined the Sharks.

CHAPTER 7

Dragon Days

Saints Behaving Badly

Without Jack Gibson's stern presence, I'm afraid I relaxed my standards a little and fitted in immediately and very easily with Saints' more relaxed culture. St George, captain-coached by the larrikin champion Graeme 'Changa' Langlands, was so different to the Roosters under the formidable and straight-laced Gibbo. When I asked my mate Keiran Speed to share his memories for this book, he didn't pull punches about my couple of years in the red and white: 'John would train at four o'clock and then by six they'd all be up the Carlton pub with vice-captain and test star Billy Smith and Langlands shouting the beers. They'd have six schooners before they went home. I mean, that was the call of the day all the time. John would match them beer for beer, no problems at all. His personality and string of jokes lit up Saints just as they had lit up the Bondi surf club, Bondi United and the Roosters before them. People were attracted to John. He was funny and charismatic and he loved a good time. I'm not saying he was a drunk, but he *could* drink and he *did* drink.'

I was still in strife with my bad knee when I turned up for pre-season training with St George. Nowadays you usually recover relatively quickly from knee operations, thanks to keyhole surgery. In 1972 they had to slice into the knee under general anaesthetic, extract the damaged cartilage, sew up the knee again, leaving a big scar, and then you'd have to convalesce with your knee elevated for a week or two and it was months before you could run again.

I could run OK, in fact I won all the distance runs at training, but my new team-mates were alarmed at my pronounced limp when I walked up stairs. 'My knee's as good as gold,' I assured them, 'I'll be right.'

I was, too. After hurting my knee again in the first trial, I recovered and had two good years at St George. The Saints' glory days were behind them then, their run of eleven straight premierships having come to an end in 1966, and Provan, Raper, Clay, Ryan, Walsh, Lumsden and King had all moved on. But in 1972 and '73 we were a good team that worried the premiership big guns such as Souths, Manly-Warringah, Cronulla-Sutherland and the Roosters. I played most matches the first year, but my second year with Saints, 1973, was a bit of a wipe-out. My knee was still dodgy and I played only a handful of games.

Lining up alongside Changa and Billy Smith were the supremely gifted 'Lord' Ted Goodwin, Roy Ferguson, Barry Beath, Col Rasmussen, Teddy Walton, Garry Pethybridge and my long-time friend Graham Bowen.

My introduction to Saints was when sixteen of us Dragons squeezed into a twelve-seater bus and headed off to the bush. We had too much to drink and I vomited all the way from Buladelah to Namorah, fair dinkum. Barry Beath, a grand forward, a truck driver and a hard worker, was the designated driver.

As bad as we behaved, it was nothing compared with Saints' legendary trip a few years previously to their sponsor Penfolds' vineyard at Minchinbury. That day Billy Smith, after sampling generous quantities of Penfolds' product, commandeered the bus while we were still at lunch and drove off. Half an hour later there was a phone call for our chairman of selectors, 'Monkey' Bill Summerill.

'Hey Monkey Bill,' said the voice on the other end, 'it's Billy. The bus has broken down.'

'What's wrong with it?' asked Summerill.

'It seems to have water in the carburettor.'

'How would you know that, Billy? You're not a motor mechanic.'

'Well, Monkey Bill,' Smithy went on, 'it's a safe bet, because I just drove the bloody thing into a lake.'

Kings of Kogarah

I liked Changa as a coach. Yes, he was one of the boys at the pub, but on the paddock he was all business, his manner short, sharp and hard. As he got older he realised that hard partying and winning footy games were mutually exclusive.

Once the team had a couple of days of mid-week rest and recreation in Wollongong before a match against Norths, who weren't performing well at that time. We figured it wouldn't matter too much if we let our hair down because all we had to do was turn up on the day to beat the Bears. We all had a few beers on the Friday night and were bussed back to Sydney on Saturday, badly hung-over. We were still much the worse for wear on Sunday when we faced Norths at Kogarah Jubilee Oval. Of course, they beat us. We dropped balls and missed tackles and ran out of puff. Our timing was stuffed.

Afterwards, Changa sat slumped in the dressing room and sighed. 'Dissa, you just can't do it,' he told me.

'Can't do what, mate?'

'Have too much to drink and play footy.'

'No, mate,' I said, 'you can't. It's either one or the other.'

Changa was disgusted with himself for letting the disaster happen. He knew he wasn't doing justice to his coaching career.

Langlands' lieutenant on and off the field was the roguish Billy Smith. Billy was a brave, tough and hugely talented halfback with a heart bigger than himself for Saints and Australia. He was also the Dragons' social secretary and he was a very, very, very social bloke. He liked a drink, Billy, and still does.

My best friend when I was a Saint was the hooker, Col Rasmussen. He had a fine sense of humour. Col was a fireman, then he joined the Taxation Department. At training, we'd all say to him, 'Hey, Razza, will you do my tax return for me, mate?' He'd shoot back, 'Sure, but it'll cost you, and don't think you won't be paying any tax!'

Col was always being bagged because he was so tight with a dollar. He'd grown up without a lot of money. Then he had the last laugh when he won the lottery.

My old mate Col died of cancer of the hip quite a few years ago. His wife Jill phoned me and said, 'You'd better get here to the hospital. Colin doesn't have long to go, and he wants to see you one last time.' I was a proud pallbearer at his funeral.

CHAPTER 8

When the Roosters Crowed

Back to Easts

After two years as a Saint I returned to Easts in 1974 aged 29. I had definitely missed the joint. Many of my old mates from earlier days were still on board, such as Arthur Beetson, Billy Mullins, Johnny Mayes (who'd returned from Manly), rugby international John Brass, and Mark Harris, who was back on deck after playing gridiron for a year with the Montreal Alouettes. Bunny Reilly had come home from the Sharks, and we'd been bolstered by Rabbitohs champions Ron Coote and Elwyn Walters. New blokes at the Roosters since my day were Wallaby Russell Fairfax, and Kevin Stevens, Greg Bandiera, Ian Mackay, Laurie Freier, Harry Cameron, Eric Ferguson and Bruce Pickett.

Best of all, though, was that Jack Gibson was back as coach after a couple of seasons at Newtown, and he had a whole new bag of tricks to add to his tried-and-tested ideology after again studying the methods and motivational ploys of the great American gridiron coaches. By now, too, he had a second-to-none support team that comprised the thoughtful, wise and football-savvy Ron Massey as his right-hand man; Mick Souter as conditioner; Alf Richards, who doubled as trainer and ambulanceman; Jack's old Roosters front-row partner Terry Fearnley as assistant coach; and Gerry Seymour, who kept the stats. Jack told me he wanted Bunny and me in his team again because he thought we were older, wiser and more experienced and could teach and inspire the young blokes in the side.

I hadn't planned to quit St George. I was looking forward to another season, one to atone for my injury-riddled 1973, when I bumped into Jack and he said, 'There's a spot for you with the Roosters. Don't suppose you're feeling homesick …' I realised that I was. Changa Langlands wasn't happy when he returned from the 1973 Kangaroo tour and learned that I'd jumped ship. He told me, 'I wouldn't have let you leave if I'd been here.' Even though my crook knee had restricted my performances, he liked having me around the place. I had a knack of contributing to a happy atmosphere.

Captain Peard

Jack shocked me – and the rugby league world – at the start of the '74 season when he named me captain over the more-fancied Arthur Beetson and the regular skipper Ron Coote. He didn't consult any of us. When we looked at the team he stuck on the wall for the opening pre-season match, the 'C' was beside my name. 'The appointment isn't permanent, nor is it temporary,' announced Jack in typically enigmatic style. 'It's been a few seasons since I was at Easts and the only players I really know are John Mayes and John Peard. I want to start off my new job with somebody I know leading the side. It's as simple as that. Naturally I thought a lot about the captaincy before I decided on Peard. Ron Coote wants to play for Australia again this season and is training enthusiastically towards this goal. I don't want to start him off as captain and then have to cut him off from the job.'

As it turned out, my shot at the captaincy *was* temporary. Arthur Beetson was soon given the job and, as history shows, he made a fine fist of it.

Success, Thanks to Gibbo

Gibbo also altered the Roosters' style of play. He had no worries about our attack, but he had serious qualms about our forwards' defence. Referring to his statistics book, he pointed out that his old team, Newtown, had no tries scored against it through the forwards in the last thirteen games of the season, while Easts' forwards leaked twenty-six. He moved Cootey from his regular cover-defending role into the front line of defence, and drilled into our heads the importance of tackling relentlessly and hard. He said that we were capable of scoring twenty points a game, which meant that if the opposition could be contained to scoring nineteen or less, then, clearly, we'd have a bloody good year.

As the 1974 season got under way I thought we'd do well, but I never dreamed we'd do as well as we did. Jack initiated us into the newfound knowledge he'd gleaned in the United States. To be honest, we thought some of his innovations were a bit strange – wearing mascara in night games to reduce glare from the lights, running backwards gridiron-style to pick up a ball-runner or 'receiver', calling the try line 'the stripe', Mark Harris with his huge hands throwing long spiral American football passes and drop-punting instead of passing. I would say to John Brass, 'This is ridiculous, it'll never work', but we did what we were told because we had total faith in Jack. And, lo and behold, some of his new moves worked a treat, maybe not next week, but a little way down the track and usually in a vital game against a gun side. Someone would call the move and we'd blow the opposition wide open. The gap would open, straight through … try!

A Memorable Decider

Just before the grand final against Canterbury-Bankstown, former Test skipper Keith Barnes came out in the press with some advice for our opposition: pound Peard and win. Well, they did, but they didn't. The Roosters came home 19–4. In the match, I got the ball about two passes wide of the ruck, pirouetted, ran backwards and completed a hand-off to Ron Coote, who passed to Mark Harris who scored the try. The successful play had a role in my realising one of my greatest childhood dreams: playing a great game in a grand final win. 'You never know,' I thought to myself, 'if this keeps up I might even play for Australia.'

Commentator Frank Hyde named me his man of the match in the triumph, Easts' first grand final win since 1945. As he wrote in *Rugby League Week*:

> Peard was *the* star of the grand final. Keith Barnes warned Canterbury that if they didn't bottle up Peard they'd be in trouble. Well, the Bulldogs didn't pay enough attention to Peard and look what happened. Peard did not make one mistake through 80 minutes of football ... Peard's name was 'lost' in the try scored by Mark Harris which was the turning point. Yet Peard was the architect of that try. It was his quick thinking which led to the initial break. Easts were leading 7–4 and on the wrong end of the penalty count when Peard darted to the right. He dummied the defence and ran to the left where he perfectly positioned Ron Coote. Peard had drawn the defence and created the gap for Coote. Coote, coming through on the burst, then set up Harris who brushed the cover out of his path. And what about Peard's defence! He surely must have topped the tackle count. And his goal kicking and line kicking were other standout features of his performance.

Jack's Magic Touch

At the end of that premiership-winning year, John Brass, a consummate centre with the best hands in the game, was asked what made Jack Gibson special. He thought a bit, then replied: 'He has instilled in me and every other member of the team a greater will to win. He has tattooed on our mind that there are no prizes for running second. Every member of the Eastern Suburbs team has Jack's drive to succeed. When you take the field you know you can't let Gibson down. If you do, you are also letting yourself down. He has my confidence. No longer do I go out and play for myself. I play for Jack, and if I play for Jack I'm playing for my team-mates and my club.'

Brassy was right. We were playing for the best coach in the business. Even today, over thirty years later, Jack's aphorisms are as fresh in my mind as if he'd said them a moment ago. 'Luck is preparation meeting opportunity …' If you supported the ball carrier, he'd turn the ball inside to you and you'd score; if you didn't you wouldn't. 'Luck never follows a stumblebum around,' said Jack.`

One of Jack's many talents was improving the strengths you had and eliminating your weaknesses. Our prop Grant Hedger couldn't use the ball to save his life, but Don Furner, Gibbo's predecessor, tried to turn him into a Beetson-like ball distributor. That was never going to work. Jack recognised that Grant was a hard-tackling, hard-running forward, period. That was his job for Jack, nothing more, and Grant performed his role to perfection.

Artie and Bunny

Arthur Beetson, under Don Furner and now Jack Gibson, had blossomed from 'Half-a-Game Artie' into an all-time great. He was fast for such a big man, and he had a step. As a ball player, he had a solid centre of gravity and hugely strong legs, hips and arms, which enabled him to lift the ball free from the attentions of gang tacklers and slip beautiful passes to supports. He was a hard man, though not as bad-tempered as when he was younger. He was brave and tough and he could tackle: the complete package. When Arthur called for the ball, we'd all get edgy –

because you were always a chance to be on the receiving end of his pass and woe betide you if you weren't ready for it. His vision was so good, he could see the gaps before they opened up and put blokes exactly in the right position to take advantage.

For all his mastery of rugby league, Arthur was a bundle of nerves before a game. It was usual for him to have a little vomit just as he was leaving the dressing room. Once he spewed up a bright red substance, and I said, 'Christ, Arthur, you're chucking blood.' He replied, 'Peardy, it's just those Cherry Ripes I ate last night.'

Arthur was inspirational, as were Brass and Coote. Any time we needed a special play or a great run or tackle, they'd deliver.

Bunny Reilly too. Like Artie, his presence on the field unsettled the opposition. He didn't have to throw punches; other players could *smell* that Bunny was tough and they'd steer clear of him. He was Jack's assassin. Before we played Manly, Jack would pull Bunny aside and say, 'Bill Hamilton, Norm Pounder, Kenny Day [Manly's hard-running forwards], they're yours.' Manly had a move in which their hooker, Fred Jones, would take a tap and give it to one of those three, who charged into the opposition. Very simple but they were powerful blokes and it worked. Bunny's job was to hit the ball-runner like a Mack truck and close him down as brutally as the rules allowed. I remember him smashing the 110-kilo Hamilton and Day, and seeing the impact hurl them high into the air.

In the Footsteps of Giants

Jack had the knack of taking the pressure off before a big game. I knew my responsibility in that '74 grand final would be heavy.

I had to spark the attack, tackle for my life and, as if that weren't enough, Jack had assigned me touch-finding and goal-kicking duties because Brassy was carrying a niggling injury. Yet in the lead-up week to the grand final, Jack's only advice to me was to make sure that when I kicked for touch, the ball went out. That's all he said. I felt I could deliver on that command, and anything else I did in the grand final was a bonus.

The night before the game he took us for a few beers at the Olympic Hotel in Moore Park Road, where years before I'd joined my mate Les Hayes in souveniring touring teams' jerseys. Then we all strolled over to the Sydney Cricket Ground and checked out the dressing rooms where the greats had changed into their footy gear and where we would be changing on grand final day. After all that, how could we not turn up ready to play?

Funny what you remember about key events in your life. My father-in-law back then had a service station in Bulldogs territory. After we qualified for the premiership decider, I gave him an Easts jumper and, brave man, he hung it over a bowser. He didn't sell much petrol that week!

Getting Some Laughs

Jack Gibson knew that a team with good morale has a better chance of performing well on the paddock than an unhappy side. Jack wanted his players and their wives and girlfriends to get along and there were many terrific social occasions we enjoyed. Our Red Faces talent quests were, however, only for the blokes. Just like during Gibbo's previous tenure at the club, everyone had to perform an act, whether it be singing, dancing, telling jokes or just wearing women's clothes, and face the judges, often Jack and Ron Massey.

I reprised my turns as Frank Hyde and Ken Howard, and added Paul Hogan's character Hoges to my repertoire. By the mid-'70s, I was a big fan of Hogan. I appreciated his dry and laconic, very Australian sense of humour. I learned to take off Hoges pretty accurately, and was always being asked to do a Hoges at Red Faces and other functions. No one had to twist my arm. I'd put on the sleeveless shirt, the Newtown footy socks, the stubbies, light up a Winfield (like Bill Clinton, I never inhaled) and reel off the jokes.

Sometimes the humour in the skits wasn't politically correct, but it was harmless enough. 'Evening, viewers,' I'd drawl. 'I came home the other night and I caught my five-year-old son playing with his testicles in the bath. "Dad," he said, "are these things my brains?" I said, "Not yet, son, not yet."'

Probably the biggest laugh I ever got had nothing to do with my jokes. Remember how Hoges would be lowered from a helicopter at the start of his TV show? Well, I'd send that up by climbing to the top of a big extension ladder that three blokes were holding steady, and diving off onto the stage with a crash.

I learned very early that I could make people laugh. I also have a terrific long-term memory – even after my stroke – and can remember jokes. I can also accurately reel off all my friends' telephone numbers without a thought.

Jack took Red Faces very seriously. Once Mark Harris failed to show up and he cancelled the entire night. It was OK if we went a little close to the bone, but Jack frowned on lewd humour. One time, Mark decided he would play a commentator of a blue movie; he turned the lights down low in the auditorium and went on and on about this couple getting it off down by a river bank. At the end of the skit the lights came on and Jack's seat was empty. He didn't say anything, just got up and left. None of us ever tried anything like that again.

I was getting a reputation as a bloke who could stand up in front of a crowd and amuse them. Some policeman friends of Ron Coote from Darlinghurst Police Station needed an MC and someone who could tell a few jokes for a function. Ron asked me if I'd do it and I happily agreed to. Afterwards the head cop presented me with a plaque that read: 'With thanks from Darlinghurst Police Station to John Peard.' I was overwhelmed and told him I'd go straight home and put the plaque on my mantelpiece. 'Don't be a fuckin' idiot,' said the policeman. 'Put it in your glove box in case a copper pulls you over for speeding!'

Another time a few years down the track the Roosters were doing some skits at Bondi surf club to raise money to buy lifesaving equipment and even though I'd left the club I dropped by to do my Hoges routine. Afterwards the players were up on the roof of the club drinking beer. For some reason I've since forgotten, I locked horns with Bob Fulton, who was Easts' coach then. We ended up wrestling and he was a very powerful guy. Bob couldn't believe I was as strong as I was. I didn't tell him I'd been lifting weights and doing wrestling training since I was a kid. Fulton and I never really saw eye to eye on the field. Him stomping on my head and splitting it wide open in an early encounter may have had something to do with that.

I was honoured to meet a real comedian in the dressing room back in '74. Phil Silvers was a veteran American jokester and movie star whose TV character, the wisecracking, double-dealing Sgt Ernie Bilko, is considered by many fans to be a comedy immortal. There I was, donning my socks and jockstrap and slapping Vaseline on my eyebrows, when I saw Phil, who was a guest of Easts' management. I crept up behind him and went, 'Grrrrrrrrr', which was a noise he made as Sgt Bilko.

Phil looked at me and said, 'Is that the best you can do, son?'

I replied, 'Yes, I've only seen your show once … and that was enough.'

Well, he broke up. Fact was, I loved Sgt Bilko and watched it every chance I got.

The Bomb and the Bomber

In 1975, my second year back at Easts, I was twenty-nine years old. I was an old man in rugby league terms. Now, suddenly, after ten years as just a sound first grader, my career, unbelievably, was about to step up a gear.

The bomb had been an integral part of rugby league since Adam played for the Eden 4 stone 7s. It was called an up-and-under then. The kick was a high punt, a towering, speculator kick put up by desperate teams who couldn't threaten the line any other way: boot it high, get under the ball and hope for the best. The up-and-under was a lottery in which anyone had a chance of grabbing the ball. In 1975 and '76 I learned how to take the speculation out of the tactic and kick so accurately that I could regularly land the ball wherever I wanted, which was usually between the opposition's try line and the dead-ball line. Two or three team-mates would be on the spot to catch the ball and score or crunch the poor defender who caught it. Gibbo rejected criticism that the bomb was a negative and boring tactic. 'It's an exciting part of play,' he insisted. 'There is no known defence. You can't fluke defence with the bomb. Only through pure skill can you manage it. You have to have skill to kick a bomb, and skill to catch one. Leave it alone.'

I practised my kicking a lot, pretty much every day for around forty-five minutes or more. I put up kick after kick at training, and even when I was supposedly off-duty, I'd go down to a park near my home at Blakehurst and kick to John Young, a fourteen-year-old who lived next door. I took half a dozen balls, each one a duplicate of the ones we played with in premiership games: a new one, an old one, a big one, a small one and a white one. I practised kicks for the line, goal kicks, stabs, grubbers, chips and, most of all, the bomb. After a while I could place any of them on a ten-cent piece, and then I began concentrating on landing the ball on the crossbar or the uprights to add another element of uncertainty.

After I learned to terrorise teams with my aerial bombardment, I was nicknamed 'Bomber'. And today, even though they would change the rules to blunt the bomb's effectiveness (the bomb defuser got to retain possession instead of having to drop-kick it back to the attacking team), the kick is an essential part of every team's armoury, with three or four players as accurate as I was.

It all happened this way. In '74 Jack Gibson invited Peter Phipps, a kicking coach from Australian Rules, to teach me, Russell Fairfax and John Brass the drop punt, an incredibly accurate kick. By poring through his books of statistics, Jack had figured out that plenty of tries came through the air. He got me positioning little chips over the top, and Russell Fairfax and, the following year, Ian Schubert, had the pace and anticipation to reach the ball on the full. I then began experimenting with kicking the ball so that it landed between the opposition try line and their dead-ball line. Kicking it high allowed a few more players time to run up and get underneath the ball. A bit of obstruction of their fullback was inevitable, and even if he did clean up, we got the ball back from their goal-line drop-out.

Jack Gibson–coached teams had in past years been accused of playing stodgy, percentage-style (though winning) footy. Jack, in my view, was making the best of the skills of the men at his disposal. There were no superstars in the Easts 1967 and '68 sides that made the semis. This was not the case at the club in 1975, when we fielded possibly the strongest club team ever, and Jack unleashed us. That year we won twenty games and were beaten just twice. Manly, who came second, had thirty competition points to our forty. We scored 469 points and only 198 were notched against us. Johnny Mayes was the season's leading try scorer with sixteen and Mark Harris was second with fourteen. Our defence was streets ahead of any other team's. In the second round we only had ten or more points scored against us in a match twice, when we beat Manly 11–10 and Wests 12–11.

Back to Back

Our grand final opponents were our old rivals and my former team-mates, the St George Dragons. For the record, our team that day, 20 September 1975, was Ian Schubert, Bruce Pickett, Bill Mullins, John Brass, John Rheinberger (plucked from lower-grade obscurity by Jack to make his first-grade debut after Mark Harris broke his leg in the final the week before), yours truly,

Monkey Mayes, Kevin Stevens, Barry Reilly, Ron Coote, Arthur Beetson (skipper), Elwyn Walters and Ian Mackay. From time to time, when best-ever grand final teams are mentioned, this team is rated by many pundits level with the great Saints teams of their golden era in the 1950s and '60s and the Rabbitohs of the late '60s and early '70s. Our opponents were Graeme Langlands, Paul Mills, John Chapman, Roy Ferguson, Ted Goodwin, John Bailey, Billy Smith, Lindsay Drake, Bruce Starkey (after Robert Stone pulled out injured), Peter Fitzgerald, Henry Tatana, Steve Edge and Barry Beath. Oddly enough, even after our great year, we were by no means confident of victory, because St George had downed us 8–5 in the major semi-final just a fortnight before. Perhaps to give us an edge, Jack put us on a high-protein, high-carbohydrate diet.

The game has gone down in rugby league folklore as 'the White Boots Grand Final'. His old Kangaroo mate Ken Irvine, who worked for Adidas, had given Graeme Langlands a pair of white boots. Nowadays players have no problem sporting white, gold, red and silver boots and no one thinks twice. Back in those more conservative times, though, anyone wearing boots of a different hue than black was considered a lair and a bighead.

If Changa had had the game of his life in that grand final, no one would remember those white boots today. Unfortunately he had a shocker. Before the game the old champion, nearing the end of his illustrious career, had an injection to kill the pain of a groin injury, but the needle missed its mark and deadened his entire leg. The first sign that anything was wrong was when he kicked in open play. Normally that kick would have gained his team fifty or sixty metres. That day it skewed crazily off his boot and went into touch about ten metres down-field. That wonderful sidestep was nullified. He had no pace. In his desperation, he made uncharacteristic errors. The game was close, 5–0 at half-time, thanks to a Johnny Mayes try after he backed up a Bruce Pickett bust. Then, when Langlands defied medical advice not to return to the field, we ran away with it. Typical was when our winger Bruce 'Veranda-head' Pickett (so named by Les Hayes because of his prominent brow) waltzed around Changa like the Saints legend was rooted to the turf to score a long-range try. At full-time the score was 38–0, and we had dealt St George the biggest shellacking in grand final history.

Apart from the scoreline that came courtesy of a spate of wonderful tries by Mayes (two), Brass (two), Mackay, Schubert, Beetson and Pickett and my seven goals, the game is memorable for a spectacular and sickening collision in the fifth minute between man of the match Ian Schubert, who had replaced Russell Fairfax at fullback after Fairy broke his leg in a mid-season Amco Cup fixture, and 'Lord' Ted Goodwin, Saints' mercurial and flamboyant centre. Teddy chipped and chased. Schuey kept his eyes on the ball. The pair collided at top speed and each reeled backwards. Our guy, who had one of the biggest and hardest heads ever seen on a rugby league player, was shaken, theirs was KO'd. Anyone who runs into Schuey's head is in trouble, I say. Ian rides a motorbike these days and he can't find a helmet large enough to fit his noggin.

After the match Artie and I tried to console our old friend Changa. He was a shattered man. Rugby league can be the cruellest of sports.

Ronny Coote, Bunny Reilly and Artie Beetson were magnificent that day. Artie dominated the Saints' forwards through his trademark combination of guile and brute force; Bunny drove blokes backwards and then dumped them; and Cootey was dynamic, making numerous incisive bursts on the edge of the rucks and tackling like a man possessed.

In the dressing sheds, Artie gave Jack a wonderful accolade. 'Thanks, Jack,' he said. 'I'll never be able to repay you for the influence you've had on my life, on and off the field. Winning two premierships on the trot is only a token payment for the time and effort you've put in. You're a coach, father and brother rolled into one.' I could only echo his sentiments.

Gibson and God

On a less reverent note, plenty of Jack jokes were doing the rounds at the victory celebrations that stretched into the following week. In one, the coach gets home late from training on a freezing night and climbs into bed beside his wife, Judy. She says, 'God! Your feet are cold.' He replies: 'Here at home, Jude, you can call me Jack.'

In another, a footy fan dies and goes to heaven. He's shooting the breeze with St Peter at the Pearly Gates when he notices a playing field inside and standing on it is a big bloke with heavy glasses holding a clipboard, smoking a Craven A, and laying down the law to a bunch of footy players. The fan asks St Peter, 'Who's that?' and St Peter replies, 'Oh, that's God. He thinks he's Jack Gibson.'

After Jack coached us to forty-three wins in forty-nine games in 1974 and 1975, God could be forgiven for getting with the strength.

CHAPTER 9

For Australia

My International Debut

The night of the 1975 grand final, we went to Ronny Coote's house at Maroubra to continue the festivities after the celebrations at the Sydney Cricket Ground. I was propping up Ron's bar when over the radio they announced the Australian team that would take on the Kiwis in the following week's World Series tournament match in New Zealand. I couldn't hear the broadcast, but Ronny came straight over, shook my hand and said, 'Congratulations, Peardy, you've made it.'

I was dumbfounded. I knew I was a chance after an excellent and consistent year, but selection at the age of thirty came as a shock. Arthur, who was captain, John Brass, Monkey Mayes,

Mark Harris, Ian Schubert and Ian Mackay also made the touring team. Ron Coote should have been picked too, but he withdrew. He would have been terrific. Former Roosters John Quayle and Jim Porter were picked from Parramatta, so the side had Jack Gibson's stamp all over it.

Dad was in the grandstand at Auckland's Carlaw Park to see me make my Test debut when we beat New Zealand. Before the match, Keith Barnes, the former great fullback for Balmain and Australia, gave me a nice rap in *Rugby League Week*:

> Peard's understanding with Arthur Beetson and John Brass will cause New Zealand a ton of trouble. Peard is the form player of 1975. Before this year he was known as a defensive five-eighth, but his attack has blossomed under Jack Gibson's tactical coaching. Peard is now a busy type of player who thinks only for the man in support. He anticipates very well and his defence is still as tenacious as before. I am sure [Test coach] Langlands will rely on Peard's tactical kicking to worry the Kiwis.

Lefts, Rights, Hooks and Uppercuts

Next challenge for the Australian selectors was to name a side to go to the Northern Hemisphere to play England, Wales and France in the remaining World Series matches. It fell to Australia's coach to announce the lucky players' names at our team hotel in Auckland after the New Zealand game. I was standing with John Quayle when Changa read the names from a sheet of paper: 'Arthur Beetson, Tommy Raudonikis, Ray Higgs, Greg Pierce, George Piggins, Terry Randall, John Rhodes ...' He came to the end of the list, and neither Quayle nor I was included.

We literally slumped onto the floor in disappointment. Changa broke into a grin. 'Come on, you two bastards, get up! Of course you're in the team.' Maybe it was his way of getting square for that grand final debacle.

Arthur Beetson reckons our game against Wales in Swansea was the most spiteful he's ever played in, and that it left the donnybrook that was the First Test in 1970 for dead. Wearing the blood-red jersey of Wales were some renowned hardheads such as the huge prop Jim Mills, hooker Tony Fisher (who was a boxing champion), Kel Coslett and Colin Dixon. In the melee that was the first scrum of the game, Dixon wheeled around and somehow got behind Arthur and grabbed him in a full nelson. Tony Fisher then took the opportunity to use Artie as a punching bag. Whack! Whack! Lefts, rights, hooks and uppercuts. Arthur wasn't impressed. Tony later gave Mick Cronin the rounds of the kitchen. Even the Welsh coach got involved in the fighting when he ran onto the field from the dugout to king-hit Ray Higgs. They won the fight, hands down, but we won the match, 18–6.

The Night I Forgot John Quayle

That wild game was the last one that John 'Canon' Quayle played on tour. I passed him the ball and he was crash-tackled by Jimmy Mills. We all heard the crack and saw his dislocated shoulder bone poking out of his back.

He was taken to hospital, operated on and given painkillers to dull his agony. When he finally showed up back at the team hotel, he was wrapped up like a mummy. 'I'm going home,' he said forlornly.

'Why?' I asked.

'I'm in terrible pain and I won't be playing any more. I just want to go home.'

'Jack, a tour of Britain and France is what every player dreams about,' I said. 'You can't go home. I'll look after you, mate. I'll be your carer. You find out who your best friends are when you can't take care of yourself.'

Next day we left for the French leg of the tour. At our hotel in Perpignan, I carefully propped up the heavily bandaged Quayle in his bed, made him comfy, fluffed his pillow, and put a book beside him where he could read it, because he was so heavily bandaged and his arms were strapped to his sides so he wouldn't move and perhaps suffer another dislocation of his damaged shoulder. Then, it being dinnertime, about 6.30 pm, I said I'd go down and get him something delicious to eat from the hotel kitchen.

Sadly, I was waylaid down in the bar by a bunch of the boys. At around 2.30 am Tommy Raudonikis asked me how the Canon was. 'Oh, shit!' I said, panic-stricken. 'I forgot all about him!'

I tore upstairs to our room to find a furious Quayle, who'd been sitting trapped on the bed, in pain and starving, for the past eight hours. 'Peard!' he snapped when I burst into the room with a packet of stale crisps. 'I'm glad you're looking after me, mate. I'd hate to see how you'd treat someone you *weren't* looking after!'

Knocked Rotten

George Piggins was another casualty of that Wales game. He was another victim of big Jim Mills. For the next week, George looked like he'd been kicked by a horse. His head was about twice its normal size. Back in his hotel room, George looked at himself in the mirror, took in the sorry sight, and turned to his room-mate, Arthur Beetson. 'Do you know what, Artie?' George said. 'That Jim Mills can't hit.'

I had to wait till a match against England to cop it. A big forward caught me with a head-high tackle and I was knocked out and carried from the field. I spent eight days in a Leeds hospital being treated for concussion. When I was released from care I returned to camp and found myself in the team to play England in a mid-week match. I was amazed that even though I wasn't fit, Changa picked me and left out Steve Rogers. I couldn't believe it because Steve was the better player. Changa always had a soft spot for me. Anyway, after the first tackle I was seeing double, sometimes triple. Changa realised something was wrong and at half-time he asked me how I was. I said, 'I think I'll be OK, but I'm seeing three balls out there.'

Replied the coach, 'Then just make sure you catch the right one!'

That World Series campaign, which we won, gave us memories to last a lifetime. We travelled to London, through England and France and down into Spain, where we saw the bullring at Pamplona. I've had a love affair with Europe ever since.

Changa Hangs Up His Boots

After a training session in Huddersfield in Yorkshire, Changa produced his infamous white boots and strung them over the crossbar. That was the last we ever saw of them. In the years since, they've gone down as legendary artefacts of rugby league and when I see Changa these days he rarely fails to grizzle, 'Jesus, I wish I'd kept those bloody boots. They'd be worth a fortune on eBay!'

On Tour

George Piggins, who in recent years waged a brave battle to ensure his beloved Rabbitohs remained in the competition, was, and is, a character. He was a rugged little hooker who trained in bare feet and became a millionaire after he invented a device to load trucks and made some astute business dealings. On the field, he took no prisoners and his battles with Mal Reilly were monumental. George was a man who was feared and respected, and with good reason.

Arthur told me that he arranged to meet Piggins in the bar one night after training but when he tried to buy George a beer, he declined. 'What's up?' said Arthur. George explained, 'Mate, I'm a teetotaller. I'm mad enough without the grog. Think how mad I'd be on it.'

Anyone rooming with Arthur Beetson was a lucky man. He was a terrific roomie. Nothing was too much trouble for him. One day George said to him, 'Arthur, you clean my boots, you keep our room tidy, you wash our clothes, you make our tea and coffee every morning. What can I do for you in return?'

'Easy, George,' replied Arthur. 'Keep that bloody Tom Raudonikis and Terry Randall out of this bloody room!'

In a tour where discipline was, shall we say, relaxed, Tommy, Terry, Ray Higgs and Graham Eadie were holy terrors. They became known as the Rat Pack. They'd wait till their team-mates had gone out, then sneak in and ransack their rooms. They'd up-end furniture, hide disgusting objects in the bedding and eat everything in the refrigerator. They were always the blokes sitting up the back of the bus or in the bar till the early hours and forever playing practical jokes. I'd like to tell you some of them, but if I did, this book could get banned or have to be distributed in a plastic wrapper.

Well, there *is* one yarn I can tell. We were all leaving our base in Leeds, the Dragonara Hotel, and the Rat Pack, who as usual were in the bar early, decided they'd ambush certain players as they came down from their rooms and exited the lift, by dousing them with pints of beer. Tommy, Terry, Graham and Ray waited by the lift door, pints poised, and – splash! – let their team-mates have it as they emerged decked out in their natty team blazer, tie and hat. Poor Johnny Rhodes copped the beer straight over his head and was soaked to the skin. Johnny, a nice, mild-mannered kind of guy, took it beautifully. 'I guess this means it's my shout, fellas?' he asked with a grin.

Then the formidable George Piggins got out of the lift. All hyped up by his great joke, 'Wombat' Eadie urged on the other Rats, 'Let's get George!' One look at the feisty expression on Piggins' face was enough to make the tricksters think twice. They soon lost their drinks and offered a lame and shame-faced, 'Oh, good morning George.' Wise move.

CHAPTER 10

Go West, Young Man

'Terry, I'm Your Man'

When I returned to Australia after the World Series I sat down with Jack Gibson and Easts' management to renew my contract for season 1976. I was a little taken aback when Jack didn't seem too pleased to see me. As an established international, I felt justified in asking for a bit more money for '76 than I'd received in '75. Jack baulked.

'How's your knee and your head?' he demanded. He said he was worried that my bad knee wouldn't hold up through the season, and feared that my concussion in England would have a lingering effect. When a boxer is knocked out, he must remain under strict medical supervision for a period before he can fight again because there's always the chance that a bleed on the brain can recur. Not rugby league players in my era. I was playing again just days after the English forward KO'd me, and I received another head-knock in my comeback match. Jack had every reason to be concerned for me, as a friend, and for his team, who could ill-afford to have a crock five-eighth.

I understood Jack's reticence to offer me the contract I requested – after all, I was thirty years of age – yet at the same time I had to do the best for myself and Christine and our daughters. I was ripe for the picking when Terry Fearnley, who had been Jack's coaching deputy at the Roosters in 1975 and had just won the first-grade coaching job at Parramatta, offered me a contract with the Eels. In fact, 'offered' is not the word. Terry put me under immense pressure to link up with him. He called me repeatedly; he came to my house. He made me feel special, and very wanted.

Terry asked what condition my knee was in and I was honest with him. I told him it was far from perfect. His reply? 'Doesn't matter. If your knee breaks down, you can teach the blokes how to kick.'

I shook Terry's hand and said, 'Terry, I'm your man.'

When I told Jack I was leaving the Roosters, he smiled and said, 'Oh, you've gone to Parramatta for the big paper bag of money, eh?' That hurt a bit. Jack knew that wasn't my way. But I guess he was a bit surprised, maybe shocked, that I had walked out.

I'm very glad to say that my parting company with Jack did not affect our friendship. We both knew that football is a hard-headed business, and appreciated each other's position. In years to come, Jack thought nothing of ringing me to tap my thoughts on a particular player his team was coming up against on the weekend. 'What's he like under pressure?' he'd probe. 'Does he step off his right or left foot? Does he pass better to one side than the other?' I was honoured that he thought so much of my opinion. Not that he ever asked me about a Parramatta team-mate. He knew better than to do that.

Once I left the Roosters I was a loyal Eel, and nothing gave me greater pleasure in my first year with the club than beating Easts three times out of three, including when we knocked them out of the comp in the preliminary final. Jack Gibson and I have been mates now for more than forty years, and my opinion of Gibbo hasn't changed. He is the most remarkable and astute man I have ever known.

It was a wrench for me to leave the Roosters, though. They were my first senior club, and with them I'd progressed from a club player to an international, and of course we'd won two comps. When you've won a premiership with a bunch of blokes – training together from the previous November, the weekly grind, the crunch matches, and the huge deciders at the business end of the season – they are special to you, and remain so for as long as you live. Opinion is divided about what's most important to a player: representing Australia, his state in State of Origin, or winning a grand final. I have no doubt that winning the premierships with the Roosters in 1974 and '75 were the highlights of my career.

Parramatta's Champions

I was joining a special group of men at Parramatta. There was Terry, who was a tremendous coach, as you'd expect given his apprenticeship with Gibbo, and a decent and honourable man. My team-mates included a fierce, talented all-international pack comprising Ray Price, Geoff Gerard, Ray Higgs, Ron Hilditch, Denis Fitzgerald and Graham Olling, and speedy and industrious backs John Kolc, Mark Levy, John Moran, Ed Sulkowicz, Neville Glover and Jimmy Porter. From the outset I proved to the boys at Parramatta that I was bloody serious. That I wasn't just hoping to cop the money and see out my career without raising a sweat. Terry Fearnley said to me, 'Peardy, you're a senior player here and I need you to set an example to the other guys.' I did my best. I won just about every training run, put in the hard work at training and in games, and spent time giving the younger blokes the benefit of my experience. They embraced me right away. A few even laughed at my jokes!

I think, looking back, that I justified Terry Fearnley's faith in me. I had a few tremendous years at Parramatta. In '76 I won a Ford Falcon for being the Rugby League's player of the year, a trip to Singapore for myself and Christine when I was honoured as *Rugby League Week*'s Player's Player of the Year. I also won *The Daily Telegraph*'s Player of the Year, and I played a role in Parra making the grand final in '76 and '77.

The Bomb Comes into its Own

My job was to be the link between forwards and backs, and to direct the team's attack. This was the year when the bomb, the accurate up-and-under that I had made a part of my armoury with Easts the year before, really came into its own. If anything, I became more accurate, and in Ray Price I had the greatest chaser of kicks who had ever played the game. Pricey made my kicks look good, because he was blessed with anticipation and determination and he chased those bombs with a single-minded and terrifying ferocity. He might get up on my left shoulder and give me a tip – say, 'Bomb the line', or 'Stick it on the twenty-five'. I'd oblige. He concentrated on that ball as it spiralled up and fell exactly where it was supposed to, and heaven help any rival who got in his way. Ray would run right through them or scramble over the top of them. He'd grab that ball and they'd be road-kill.

Ray scored twelve tries from my bombs in 1976. In one match against St George, I had to feel sorry for the red-and-whites. They scored three brilliant, length-of-the-field tries with the ball sweeping through multiple sets of hands. We scored three tries, too, all from bombs fifteen metres out from their line. A penalty sealed the game for us. As I said, rugby league isn't always fair.

In time, the bomb became Parramatta's main strike weapon. We were accused of negativity. Having sussed out where the opposition was, I would call the shots. Tell the forwards to take the ball up one-out, till we got near the opposition's quarter line, then I'd call for the ball as first receiver from the dummy half and boot it high. Our blokes would time their chase to arrive at exactly the instant the ball landed. They'd catch it themselves or smash the opposition fullback or winger and often regain possession from a goal-line drop-out. As Jack used to say, 'There's no defence against the bomb.' Every time it goes up, if the kick and chase are good, you have a fifty–fifty chance of retrieving it in a try-scoring position. My bomb was a weapon of mass destruction, and a wonderful way to pressure the opposition.

In later years, the bomb's effectiveness was defused when it was ruled that the defending team, having caught the ball on the full over their line, retained possession with a tap on the quarter line. But back in '76, it was a lose–lose situation for any team on the receiving end of a bomb. And I rained 'em down. How come other blokes weren't as effective as me? I can only put it down to a little natural kicking talent, experience, which gave me the ability to read the game and unleash a bomb at the most appropriate time … and practice, practice, practice.

The Power of the Boot

Kickers ruled in that era. If you kicked the ball out any way other than on the full in the opposition half you got the scrum feed and the put-in. That wasn't an ironclad guarantee you'd get the ball back because scrums were contested then, unlike today, but the chance was that you would, and that made rugby league a real kick-fest for a time. In the grand final against Manly at the Sydney Cricket Ground that year, I called for the ball within the first ten minutes and reefed it from the cricket pitch mound. It found touch ten metres out from Manly's line. The scrum went down. We won the ball. Kolc was tackled. Dummy half Higgs shot it to me. I bombed Manly winger Tom Mooney. Our Jimmy Porter (who knew it was coming) out-jumped Tommy and scored near the sideline. I converted. Parramatta 5, Manly 0. The power of the boot.

I delighted in terrorising other teams, and tried to give rival fullbacks a day they'd rather forget. In a semi against Saints in '76, their young fullback, Tony Quirk, dropped two of my bombs and we scored both times and ran away to a 31–6 win.

When I had my stroke I was lying in my hospital bed and a visitor arrived. He looked vaguely familiar. It was Tony Quirk, come to give me his best wishes. That's rugby league, and rugby league men, for you.

Marked Man

Inevitably, when we started winning game after game on the back of my pinpoint kicking, I became a marked man. Every match I was belted in the back play. Higgsy and Pricey were my designated minders, but they couldn't be everywhere. Even St George's tiny halfback, Mark Shulman, whacked me. The biggest beating I took was at the hands of Manly in a 1976 semi-final. My old World Series team-mate Terry Randall, who played in Manly's second row, thumped me, then Alan Thompson, Ian Martin and Bob Fulton. Martin got me again shortly after, and left my face a bloody mess. I'd always said I was a lover, not a fighter. Ray Higgs got square when he kicked Martin in the leg and the five-eighth was forced off the field with a huge cut. Manly's aggressive tactics backfired because we received a constant flow of penalties that ensured we played the game in their half, and I ended up with six goals in our 23–17 win.

Not Good Enough

We were in the grand final. My third in three years. The Seagulls regained their composure and lined up against us in the premiership decider. We were favourites, and especially so after Jim Porter scored from my bomb early on, but Manly won 13–10 thanks to Graham Eadie's five goals from six attempts.

With twelve minutes to go and Manly ahead by three, John Moran drew the Manly defence and sent a perfect pass to our unmarked winger Neville Glover. Neville dropped the ball. In desperation as the closing minutes ticked away we tried a 'flying wedge', where Ron Hilditch took the ball from a tap close to Manly's line and the other forwards virtually picked him up and drove him towards the try line like a human battering ram, but Eadie dived at Hilditch's oncoming legs and the wedge collapsed centimetres short. Game over. Higgs was magnificent for us, in spite of being knocked to the ground by Terry Randall, but Eadie's boot and the wiles and power running of Fulton and the Seagulls' English trio of Steve Norton, Phil Lowe and Gary Stephens were too much for us on the day.

I felt sorry for Terry Fearnley, for my team-mates, and for the fans of Parramatta. No team could ever wish for better supporters than the fanatical, noisy, unbelievably one-eyed Blue and Gold Army who turned up at training in their thousands and waited to cheer us when we emerged from the dressing room after a game. I believed we were a better team than Manly, but it just wasn't our day.

After the game I exchanged jerseys with Bob 'Bozo' Fulton, who was playing his last game with Manly before moving to the Roosters. I still have that mud-spattered number 4 jumper. I might donate it to the Rugby League Hall of Fame or to the Manly club to auction for charity one day. I admired Bob's footballing skills enormously – he was the best five-eighth I ever faced – but his intensity and ruthless professionalism made him a nightmare to play against. Bozo was a niggler and a pest par excellence.

I can't remember ever really getting the better of Bob on the field, but I take my revenge when I do my stand-up comedy routine. I'm always taking pot shots at Bob's reluctance to part with a buck. God, he was tight with his money. 'Oh, Bozo,' I'll say, a fond smile creasing my face. 'I remember him. He was the bloke with the reach impediment ...'

TV star

Being a close team enabled us to put our disappointment behind us and focus on going one better in 1977. Every Thursday night we'd get together at the Parramatta Leagues Club and have a bit of a do with party pies and a few beers, then we'd go down to where the bands were playing and have a dance with our wives and girlfriends.

Four of us – Johnny Kolc, John Baker, John Mann and me – represented Parramatta on Channel 10's *Rugby League New Faces*. All the teams were invited to send along their funniest blokes, or someone who could sing a bit. I found a loud chequered suit for Kolcy, who was going to tap-dance; I'd do my Hoges act; Mann (in drag) would be Delvene Delaney; and Bakes would play Strop. We had a few beers at the leagues club to get our courage up and go over our act.

Johnny Baker was perfectly cast as Strop, because he spoke a hundred miles an hour out of the side of his mouth. We called John 'Mumbles' because we couldn't understand a word he was saying. I was prepared. I wrote out Bakes' lines on a piece of paper and stuck it with sticky tape on his wrist. This is what he had to say: 'Hey Hoges, how long have you been wearing that corset you had on in the dressing room the other day?' My reply was: 'Ever since the missus found it in my glove box.' But because John tended to speak too fast and mumble his words,

I added a reminder at the end of his lines: 'PS: TAKE YOUR TIME!'

As we neared the TV station I thought we'd better rehearse. 'OK, Strop, let's hear your lines.'

Bakes began: 'Hey Hoges, how long have you been wearing that corset you had on in the dressing room the other day? PS: TAKE YOUR TIME!'

'My God,' I said, 'let's go back to the club and get on the piss ...'

But everything turned out all right on the night, as they say. We won the talent quest. We landed a $5000 voucher each for international air fares. I gave mine to an elderly couple, Parra fans who'd never been anywhere in their lives.

In Pain Against Bath's Babes

I was struggling with a damaged groin. At Christmas I was in the weights room at Parra and while doing some exercises designed to strengthen my abdominal muscles I felt a twinge of pain. Thinking nothing of it, I continued. Afterwards I was stiffer than I had ever been. What I'd done was tear the muscle in the base of my stomach away from my pubic bone. The pain grew worse with every match. Towards the end of the season it was hopeless. I played in agony. To try to alleviate the pain I would whack on heat packs and rub warming liniment deep into my groin. I could just about get through a match, but afterwards I'd be in awful pain. I soon dreaded hearing the full-time siren because I knew what was in store for me when the damaged muscles cooled down. I literally couldn't move. I couldn't get in and out of cars, I couldn't raise my legs, and once in bed, I had to stay in that position all night long. Each week, against my better judgment, I backed up for another game and more punishment. That's how much I loved playing rugby league.

St George took over from Manly-Warringah as our nemesis in '77. We had a ton of respect for them because they had one of the great forward coaches in the knowledgeable Harry Bath and a gutsy team of young goers. Craig Young, Rod Reddy, Robert Stone, Bruce Starkey, John Jansen, Steve Edge (who would become one of Parramatta's greatest servants), Robert Finch, Graham Quinn, Rod McGregor, Mark Shulman – 'Bath's Babes', they called them. Under coach Bath, Saints' forwards ran brilliant angles, used the ball well, utilised decoy runners years before anyone else, and were as hard-nosed as their mentor had been.

We lost only three of our competition games, although significantly, one of those defeats, a right thrashing, was dealt to us by a twelve-man St George side after Ted Goodwin was sent off early in the game. As minor premiers and with the game's leading goal kicker, Mick Cronin, having joined us, we were favourites to win the comp. Parra were the pick of the experts because of our consistent form, and the sentimental favourites too because in our thirty years in the premiership we had never won a grand final.

Bashed to Defeat

As it happened, Saints beat us in the major semi to be first into the premiership decider. We came back to qualify and the stage was set for one of the most dramatic grand final sagas in league history. They were the younger, faster dashers who played with seat-of-the-pants flair and raw aggression. We were older, a bit slower, more programmed, more in control of our emotions; and with me and Mick Cronin, we were thought to be superior kickers. Not that I should have even played at all in the grand final. I'd done some further damage to my bad groin in the semi, and in the grand final ran on from the bench when the game was well under way.

At half-time the score was 9–0 to Saints after they had run and tackled – and, it has to be said, bashed us – with more gusto. Three second-half goals by Cronin brought us to 9–6; then in the seventy-seventh minute, Cronin passed to Price, who swerved and sent the ball inside to centre Ed Sulkowicz who scored. If Mick could convert, the premiership was ours. He took his time, seemingly an age, to line the ball up. He stepped back, moved in, made contact and the ball skewed away.

At 9–9, this was the first-ever drawn grand final. After twenty minutes of extra time, punctuated by frantic stabs at field goals by exhausted players, the score remained the same. The match would have to be replayed.

Everyone expected the grand final replay (in which I played, even though my injured groin was giving me indescribable hell) to be a tight, controlled match like the first grand final, with little or nothing in it at the end. But Harry Bath, the wily old fox, ensured that didn't happen, by coming up with a tactic designed to put us off our game.

From the kick-off, St George turned on the biff. Stone, Young, Jansen and Reddy simply belted us out of the game. Rod Reddy was a particular offender – he was cautioned three times in the first ten minutes for punching Price, scragging him and pulling his hair. Price and Olling looked as though they'd gone twelve rounds with Joe Frazier. Saints' aggression distracted us, and our game plan went out the window.

Having won the fight, the Saints played football, and after leading 7–0 at half-time, they ran out 22–0 winners. Harry Bath had countered my kicking game by having his fastest man, Mark Shulman, race at me the moment our bloke played the ball, thereby cutting down the time I had to catch and get a good kick away. He was like a bloody cattle dog the way he harassed me. Particularly galling for me was when the scrum screwed and I lost sight of the ball in the forest of arms and legs, and their big second-rower Robert Stone picked it up and ran forty metres to score. After the match, there were rumours that St George had found a second wind during the game by vowing to avenge their halfback Mark Shulman, who had been kneed. Being younger, they seemed to cope better with the gruelling physical and emotional demands of playing another grand final.

I'd like to dispel a myth. The story is told that Terry Fearnley and Ray Higgs had a monumental argument at half-time after Fearnley refused to allow him and his fellow forwards to fight Saints' fire with fire. Not true. I was there in the dressing room at half-time, and I can state that no such brouhaha ever happened. Terry was an old forward himself who played with Jack Gibson and he was a pragmatist. I believe if he, or the forwards, felt that victory could have been gained by fighting, they would have accommodated the Dragons by turning on a hell of a stink. When you're behind 7–0, punching and conceding penalties aren't going to win you the game. Tries and goals were our only chance and we were unable to score them. Simple as that.

Battling on

The following year, 1978, I turned thirty-two, and had had an off-season operation on my groin. It never did come right. I couldn't train, which took away a lot of the enjoyment I got from the game. After training, my damaged groin would be so sore I couldn't move for hours. I was like a cripple. I went to an acupuncturist and a chiropractor, to little avail. Finally, Parramatta's team doctor, Dr Peter Manollaras, prescribed a course of cortisone injections and, apart from making me feel like a pin cushion, they relieved the pain.

My chronic groin problem prevented me from playing, of course, and while I was sitting on the sidelines for the first eight weeks of the competition I had my series of needles. Twelve weeks into the comp I was pronounced fit to play. I made it through the matches, though was never at my physical peak, and after every game I had to sit packed in ice while the other guys partied.

Meanwhile, the team was doing well, and we were everyone's pick to finally win a premiership. Mick Cronin was unbelievable that year. Maybe to make amends for missing the kick that would have won us the premiership the previous year, he scored a massive 282 points for Parramatta. When you add the points he'd also notched for City, New South Wales, and Australia on the Kangaroo tour, he accumulated a whopping 547 points, including a record twenty-six consecutive goals.

Once more, the finals were dramatic, and once more we failed when it mattered. Not that it was all our fault. Our minor semi-final against Manly ended – you wouldn't believe it – in a 13–13 draw.

Talk about déjà vu. The replay was a horror story for us. In the eleventh minute, referee Greg Hartley sent off our best forward, Ray Price (Ray was later exonerated by the judiciary). I tapped the ball forward and dived on it over the Manly line to score a try, but Hartley disallowed it, saying my foot hadn't connected with the ball when it bloody-well had. Hartley, the little bloke who insisted on running onto the field before the players at the start of a game, who posed theatrically when he made decisions, who took spectacular and attention-grabbing tumbles, and who had made his name making life a living hell for the great Artie Beetson, then awarded Manly's Steve Martin a match-winning try on the seventh tackle! To rub it in, on three occasions, he had awarded us five tackles instead of our allotted six.

One Last Season

I was gutted at the loss and in agony with my bad groin – which I knew, no matter how much cortisone I pumped into it, was never going to come right. The old body wasn't what it used to be. But it was desperately hard to walk away from a game that had been my life since I was a boy. What the hell would I do? What job would give me the chance to do something I loved in front of wonderful fans week after week? I couldn't think of one, so I saddled up again for season 1979. I was thirty-four years of age, getting on for a back.

My last year as a player was one in which I could only play occasionally. My groin continued to give me merry hell. I was in pain and I had trouble running and kicking, so I concentrated on defence, and was proud of the way I contained my rivals when I was able to get onto the paddock.

The last match I ever played in was a semi-final at the Sydney Cricket Ground against Canterbury-Bankstown. I marked Garry Hughes, a clever five-eighth but hardly a noted speedster, and Garry ran rings around me. Jack Gibson was at the game and he gave me a look that said far more than a thousand words. That look, one that betrayed his concern and exasperation, said, 'Bomber, give it away.'

I had played 199 senior games of rugby league, for Australia, New South Wales, City, Easts, St George and Parramatta in a fourteen-year career. I'd played for my country eight times, and made three international tours in the green and gold. As hard, and heartbreaking, as it was to walk away from a game that had been so close to my heart since childhood, I knew at last that it was time to get on with the rest of my life.

CHAPTER 11

Coach Peard

'Get Ready to Be Lonely'

Terry Fearnley fell on his sword at the end of season 1979. He thought that, after coming so desperately close twice but not delivering the title Parramatta so desperately wanted, he'd been head coach long enough and the club needed a change. In January 1980, with Terry's blessing, the club's board called me and asked if I was interested. Was I ever! As I knew I would, I was having trouble adjusting to life after league. I couldn't play any more, but surely after soaking up the gospel of rugby league according to Jack Gibson, Graeme Langlands and Terry Fearnley I was well equipped to take the coach's clipboard.

The Parramatta hierarchy were delighted when I signed on. I suppose I'd made a positive impression on them, and on Terry, in my playing days there. I was Terry's lieutenant. He consulted me and knew I would carry out his instructions to the letter. However, I was left in no doubt that the club expected no less from me than a premiership. The district was sick of following an also-ran rugby league team. Nothing less than premiership glory in 1980 would satisfy the people of Parramatta. I realised I would not be given a second chance at success.

I felt I had the respect of the players. At least I hoped I did. One of the hardest things for a young bloke who becomes a coach right after his playing days are over is making his charges forget that he's a mate and a peer and that he is the bloke who calls the shots. So I came in determined not to be one of the boys. I had devised a coaching philosophy based on discipline, defence, programmed attack and setting and achieving goals. I was very firm about that.

Almost from the outset I put noses out of joint. A young fullback with a shock of blond hair and an amazing array of skills had joined Parramatta from Wagga in 1978 and after paying his dues in the lower grades was now ready for first grade. I thought this bloke would be a better halfback than a number 1. I wanted him closer to the action where his extraordinary vision and feel for the game, his wonderful passing, kicking and running could be better utilised. His name was Peter Sterling.

One night at pre-season training, I pulled him to one side. 'Peter,' I said, 'get used to feeding the scrum because you're our new halfback. You won't be playing anywhere but half as long as I'm coach here.'

Amazingly, in light of what Sterlo would go on to achieve, his selection at halfback angered many of the players. It meant that two good friends of mine in Johnny Kolc and Graham Murray, both fine halfbacks, would be ousted from their specialist position; and their supporters in the team such as Geoff Gerard and especially Ron Hilditch, who loved running off Kolc and Muzza (now coach of the North Queensland Cowboys and the New South Wales State of Origin team), thought I had rocks in my head. Time proved that I didn't.

I was in hot water with Arthur Beetson as well. I didn't believe we could have two ball players – in him and fellow veteran Bob O'Reilly – in the same side. I wanted to leave the ball distribution to Bob and have Arthur, who could still raise a good head of steam and unload when he forced his way through a gap, running off him. Arthur felt I was monkeying with his game, and at thirty-five he was too old to change his style. I may have been wrong, but I believed I was right and I stuck to my decision despite Arthur and others in the team and in administration resenting it. Unfortunately Arthur spent a bit of time in reserve grade that year. I just kept reminding myself of something else Vince Lombardi, the American gridiron coach who inspired Jack Gibson in so many ways, said long ago: 'A leader needs to separate himself from his followers ... Get ready to be lonely. When your position changes, some relationships will, too. Part of being a good leader is accepting the distance that this brings.' I know Arthur was unhappy, and the way I treated him still rankled him enough for him to give me a little serve in his autobiography, *Big Artie*, but I'm glad to say we remain the best of friends.

Taking a leaf from Gibbo's book, I put an enormous amount of time into formulating my coaching philosophy. No less a master than Jack was my role model when I took on the unforgiving role of coach.

Pearls of Wisdom

Recently, when I was accumulating the material for this book, I came across some sheets of paper on which I'd scribbled a few notes, pearls of wisdom I'd worked out for myself, or read about. In my time as the Eels' coach I unloaded these truisms on my blokes. I can still remember the likes of Mick Cronin, Bob O'Reilly, Peter Sterling, Steve Ella, Eric Grothe, Ray Price, Brett Kenny and Arthur Beetson in the sheds while I came across like Winston Churchill ...

- The key to success in life and sport is knowing how to take on board good advice we receive and to reject the bad.
- Eliminate the fear of failure, which makes us scared to take on new challenges. When you make mistakes, as you inevitably will, learn from them.
- Success is the progressive realisation of worthwhile, carefully thought-out goals. Decide the right goals for you and then establish priorities in your life so you may achieve them. Let nothing deter you.
- Positive thinkers win, negative thinkers lose. Develop a positive mental attitude.
- Motivate yourself through knowing your needs and desires. Motivation involves expectation and belief and action. But recognise that while you can be motivated by fear, incentive and attitude, the latter is the only factor that can change you internally.

I studied the words of motivator Paul J Meyer. His subject was desire.

> What is desire? Desire is the vital essence of a champion's inner self. Desire is the quality that makes winners ... A man with activated desire isn't nearly as afraid of losing as a loser is secretly afraid of winning. A man with desire makes commitments; other people make promises. Desire makes a man go through a problem; other people go around them ... Desire gives a man the courage to say, I'm good, but not as good as I should be.'

The Lombardi Rules

I also made a lightning visit to the United States, to study, as Jack Gibson had done, the methods of the gridiron coaches. I was a guest of the teams from San Diego, Atlanta, Dallas and Hawaii. I met the great coach Tom Landry, another who had impressed Gibbo, and brought home suitcases stuffed with motivational tapes and books. Among the latter was a booklet that would become my Bible for football and life: *The Lombardi Rules*, written by Vince Lombardi Jr, comprising twenty-six lessons from his father, Vince senior, regarded as the greatest gridiron coach who ever lived. Lombardi coached the Green Bay Packers from 1956 to '67, taking (much as Jack did) a team of blokes used to losing, and transforming them into a championship team in just two years. The Packers won the NFL title in 1961, 1962 and 1965 and Super Bowls in '66 and '67.

I learned the Lombardi rules and applied them to my coaching at Parramatta and later at Penrith, and to every aspect of my life in the years since. They've stood me in good stead throughout my battle to survive my stroke.

Lombardi's credo is summed up in two wonderful quotes. When I read them I felt like he was talking straight to me. 'Mental toughness,' said Lombardi, 'is many things and rather difficult to explain. Its qualities are sacrifice and self-denial. Also, most importantly, it is combined with a perfectly disciplined will that refuses to give in. It's a state of mind – you could call it character in action.' Also, if you believe in yourself, he preached to his players, 'and have the courage, the determination, the dedication, the competitive drive, and if you are willing to sacrifice the little things in life and pay the price for the things that are worthwhile', anything can be achieved.

Vince Lombardi gave me a credo to live by. Reading his wisdom I came to know that honest and deep self-knowledge is a key to success. It helps you identify accurately your strengths and weaknesses and make the necessary adjustments and improvements. I came to learn by failure and hardship and that every experience, good or bad, has something to teach us. Another Lombardi lesson is to have heroes, emulate their deeds – but choose them wisely.

Lombardi taught that goals must be anchored in conviction and closely linked to what you seek to achieve. Oddly enough, some players had problems with goal setting. Peter Sterling once complained that he didn't know what he would do if he set a goal and failed to meet it. The answer is to re-align your sights to a more realistic goal and then go hard for it. I believe that goals are as essential to us as oxygen and food. I also believe that my lack of firm goals at the time contributed to my stroke in 2002.

Lombardi inspired those around him with his own high level

of commitment. 'When leaders go the extra mile,' he said, 'their troops will follow.'

He also preached that talent alone is not enough. A person with great natural ability but poor commitment will come a cropper because of 'inattention, inconsistency and laziness'. He would have agreed with Jack Gibson that discipline helps you make the tough decisions, endure pain and retain focus despite pressure and fear.

Nothing great is easily achieved, wrote Lombardi, and sacrifices are part of any successful scenario. And once you've achieved, be proud (after all, success breeds confidence and rightly so), but don't let your pride and ego obscure the truth.

He knew that a team is most effective when it plays to the strengths of its members and a wise coach tailors his game plan to take advantage of his charges' abilities. Having always been a team man, I glowed when Lombardi decreed that the best people put their team's interests ahead of personal ambitions. A good coach, too, is not a dictator, he is a delegator; he explains his strategies clearly, starting with the why and not the how. He accepts praise, but also the knocks when deserved.

Most importantly, to me at least, was when Lombardi wrote: 'Never give in. It's easy to do well when there is no pressure or stress, but how many of us can be poised when defeat is nipping at our heels? Mental toughness is not rigidity in the face of adversity; it's stability and poise in the face of challenge.'

Do or Die

I reckoned we would do well if I could instil even a fraction of the Lombardi ethos into my players, get them fit, make them disciplined, hone their skills and help them decide on, and then achieve, their goals.

I had a wonderful team and I regret today that, being a novice coach, I was not able to get the best from them in spite of my busting a gut to do so.

The second-grade coach was Mick Alchin, a very astute man who had been a fiery winger for Wests in his day. He was always suggesting young blokes he thought would make the grade in the firsts. Usually I took his advice. I was not, however, convinced that one of his charges, a lanky five-eighth named Brett Kenny, was the goods. It took me a while to realise that Mick was right and promote Brett, who of course went on to be an all-time great and was responsible for much of the glory that would come the way of Parramatta, New South Wales and Australia in the years to come.

I wish I was able to tell you that Parramatta won the comp in 1980 and delivered the premiership the district so coveted. Things didn't happen that way. The crunch match for us was the last game of the premiership rounds, against St George at our home ground, Cumberland Oval. If we won, we were in the semi-finals, if we lost, we were history. Simple as that. The district went crazy in anticipation of a big victory and the old ground was jammed on game day. We went down 20–11.

We had played well during the year, certainly been competitive, and had a number of fine wins. But we missed the semis by a point. Good, Peardy, in your debut year, but no cigar.

I learned later that Reg Sheargold, who was secretary/manager of Parramatta Leagues Club and Mick Cronin's father-in-law, and so a very influential man, addressed the committee and said, 'Look, we're cashed up, the leagues club is doing well, we can afford to hire the best coach in the business.' I was replaced at the end of the season by Jack Gibson. The rest is history: he won the grand finals of 1981, '82 and '83 and created a new super-team from the mix of up-and-comers and veterans I'd coached in 1980.

Chocolate Soldiers

Jack asked me to be his assistant coach, but I needed a break. I turned down his offer and in 1981 took a year off from coaching, a year right away from the game.

Then Charlie Gibson, Penrith's footy boss, got me on the phone. He offered me the first-grade coach's job with the Penrith Panthers for 1982 and '83. I was refreshed and champing at the bit to get back into the game I loved, so I said yes. There were times in that next two years when I wished I hadn't.

Our first training run set the tone for my time with the Panthers. I organised a run for the players up Heartache Hill in the Blue Mountains ... and I won. I was thirty-seven and had a crook groin. As I raced past the stragglers and hit the lead I heard one young bloke gasp, 'Who was that?'

His mate replied, puffing badly, 'Bloody hell! It's the coach!'

In the weights room I could out-lift anyone, even the biggest forwards. It was pretty evident I'd have to work on their fitness and strength.

The Chocolate Soldiers, as we were known (because of our brown jerseys, not because we melted when the opposition applied the heat), didn't trouble the premiership front-runners in either year. We had a fair team. No real stars but solid blokes, and there was a bit of character: the speedy fullback and winger Kevin Dann, my old Parramatta mate Mark Levy, Brett Lobb, Rob Wright, a hot young five-eighth and centre named Brad

Izzard, Ross Gigg and nippy Aboriginal halfback Henry Foster in the backs; and a tough, workmanlike bunch of forwards in Royce Simmons, Warren Fenton, Lew Platz, Darryl Brohman, Lou Zivanovic, Brad Waugh, super-coach of the future Tim Sheens (I taught him everything he knows – just joking, Sheensy!) and back-up hooker Jamie Jones. Jamie was the toughest bloke in the squad. He and Brad Waugh hit like sledgehammers and Lou always had plenty of petrol in the tank.

The best player in the side was our huge-hearted hooker Royce Simmons, who would become a Kangaroo and Panther great. When our regular captain, Tim Sheens, wanted to step down to concentrate on his business I had no qualms about replacing him with Royce, who was a leader of men on and off the field.

I was instrumental in signing up Leeton lad Chris Houghton, though I nearly stuffed it up. The plan was that I'd hand him a contract right after he played in his regional grand final. My plane from Sydney landed at Leeton about midday on Sunday. I told the taxi driver, 'Take me to the grand final. And tell me, what's Leeton like? Are they a better team than their opponents?'

The cabbie came back: 'Definitely. They're taller, and better in the air.'

'Hang on, mate. What are you talking about? Where are you taking me?'

'To the Aussie Rules grand final.'

'Hey, pal, stop the cab. I want to go to the *rugby league* grand final. Take me there, and step on the gas!'

'Mate,' said the driver, 'this cab ain't a time machine. The league grand final was *last* Sunday!'

Big Darryl Brohman was as funny then as he is today as a radio commentator and guest speaker. He reckons he was rugby league's original three-time loser. 'I played for Penrith when they hardly won a game,' he says. 'I made State of Origin but lasted only a few minutes because Les Boyd broke my jaw. And I've got the smallest dick in rugby league.'

Charlie Gibson was the brains behind Penrith paying a huge amount of money for Tony Darcy, a young Wallaby rugby union prop. Tony was a lovely chap, a well-spoken gentleman and a fine rugby union player. He struggled with the intricacies of his new code. Rugby union apologists are always shooting off their mouths about how their game is too complex for league converts; well, the same applies, believe me, for union blokes who switch to league. The pace of the game, the collisions and the one-on-one defensive workload, using the ball ... Tony knew it would take him time to come to grips with it all. Charlie Gibson, however, didn't want to appear to have bought a dud. Soon after Tony came to Penrith I arrived at training and there was Charlie, a man in his fifties who had never played league at an elite level, in his business suit, a cigarette dangling out of the corner of his mouth, schooling Tony in forward play. I thought, 'I'm getting out of here!'

I went to see Jack Gibson at his home and asked him, 'Jack, what am I going to do with this team? Can you give me any tips?'

He paused for a while and then said, 'I think your biggest problem is that you're not being allowed to run the show.'

'What can I do about Charlie Gibson?'

Jack thought again, then said in his inimitable way, 'I'm thinking about doing something about him myself.'

'What?'

'I'm thinking about ringing him up and getting him to change his surname,' drawled Jack. 'He's giving us Gibsons a bad name.'

A Fine Line

There's no use gilding the lily. As coach of Penrith I was unsuccessful. We finished third last in the comp in '82 and fourth last in '83. It was a shock to a bloke who had become used to winning. I took refuge in humour. What's the old adage? If you can't laugh you go insane. Then and later in my life when talking about the underachieving Panthers I hid my hurt with a smile.

> 'In my first month at Penrith we lost four games in a row,' I'd say, then pause … 'And *then* we went into a slump!'

> I can remember my first day on the job at Penrith like it was yesterday. And if it was tomorrow, I'd piss off tonight!

> How do I sleep when I'm coach of Penrith? Like a baby. I wake up every two hours and bawl.

I'd also tell the story of how I was stopped for speeding by a cop on my way to Penrith from Cronulla. 'Where do you think you're going in such a hurry?' asked the policeman.

'Sorry, officer,' I said, 'I'm late for training. I coach the Panthers.'

'Then on your way. You've got enough problems without me booking you!'

Before a match against the Sharks I was worried that the motivational message I'd recorded for my blokes hadn't soaked in, so I gathered them around the boot of my car, where I kept my tape recorder, and I played the tape. Imagine seventeen burly footballers in their shorts, boots and jerseys, all greased up, clustered around an open boot listening intently. Just then a Sharks fan strolled by and quipped, 'Fellas, don't buy it, it's hot!'

Seriously, though, I did a lot of soul-searching then, and subsequently I've thought long and hard about those two gruelling years. I like to believe that I didn't fail personally in my stint with the Panthers. I put an enormous amount of effort into that job, even down to recording individual goal-setting tapes for each player, and I didn't feel inferior to any coach in the game with the exception of Jack Gibson. It's a fine line between success and failure. We lost a number of games by very narrow margins. I don't think I'd have done anything differently, and that I did the best I could with the personnel and the administrative set-up at my disposal.

Flights of Fancy

Rugby league was my passion as a coach as it had been when I was a player. I thought deeply about the game and ways to make it a better spectacle. At the end of 1983, Greg Mitchell, an executive of the Australian Rugby League who is now general manager of the Parramatta Eels, sat down with me to nut out a blueprint for change in rugby league. We knew our ideas were radical, but hoped they would be food for thought to streamline the code and help it meet the challenges that would be presented by rugby union, AFL and soccer.

Among our proposals was a plan to make the game more attack-oriented to give spectators plenty of thrills and offer fans a product that was entertaining, skilful and competitive, and more than capable of holding its own against the rival codes. To that end, we advocated increasing athleticism, speed and skill levels in handling, running, tackling, passing and kicking and support play, and refining players' tactical awareness.

We proposed eliminating scrums and reducing the number of players in a team to ten (but with five replacements who could be introduced to the game from the bench at any time), to give more attacking space. The makeup of a team would be: one fullback, two wingers, two centres, five midfielders. The midfield could comprise three big, mobile men, perhaps a halfback and a five-eighth. Because of the space created, there would be less gang tackling and more one-on-one defence. (A random study of several games in 1983 indicated that 74 per cent of all tackles were effected by two or more players.) This would result in quicker play and faster clearing of the ball from the ruck. A 'yardage official' to police the five metres in the ruck would assist the referee. The advantage rule would apply when the ball was knocked on, to eliminate stoppages and promote flow of play.

From a ball out of play over the sideline, the team responsible for putting it out would lose possession, and the non-offending side would restart play with a play-the-ball ten metres in from touch, adjacent to where the ball went out. And from a ball going out on the full, the non-offending side would play the ball on the mark where it was kicked out. Also, where a player was held up or lost the ball in the in-goal area, the non-offending side would restart play with a goal-line drop-out.

We concluded by pointing out that the credibility of rugby league was our number one priority. Change in the game had been neglected. Changes did not need to be regarded as 'tough decisions' if they were considered, well planned and had the good of the game as their intention. 'What has been presented here,' we wrote, 'is a sincere attempt to upgrade rugby league as an entertainment form by changing aspects of the game that do its credibility greatest harm.'

Our radical masterplan, with its call for fewer players, the elimination of scrums, a yardage official and a steady flow of replacements, was all a bit much for its day, and none of our proposed changes was implemented. I suppose there are echoes of our blueprint in rugby league and rugby union Tens and Sevens competitions. But take a close look at the way rugby league is played today and you'll see elements of Greg Mitchell's and my reforms in the modern game, such as non-contested scrums, touchies advising the ref if teams are creeping offside, and the use of an interchange bench. In addition, the players today are multi-skilled, generally more so than players of my era.

State of Origin

I coached the Sydney City Origin sides in 1983, '84 and '85, then in 1988 I got the call to take on one of the most demanding and unforgiving jobs in Australian sport. I was asked to coach the New South Wales State of Origin team, probably thanks to my friendship with former team-mate and 1975 World Series roomie John Quayle. Canon had gone on to become general manager of the Australian Rugby League and had obviously forgiven me for shamefully neglecting him after he'd dislocated his shoulder against Wales.

Unfortunately, New South Wales were pitted against a very hot bunch of cane toads that year – Wally Lewis, Mal Meninga,

Peter Jackson, Gene Miles, Bob Lindner – and in spite of us having some fine players, including Peter Sterling, Steve Roach, Steve Mortimer and Steve Folkes, we went down in all three games: 26–18, 16–6 and 38–22.

For the first match we stayed at Sydney's Camperdown Travelodge. We trained at the oval at nearby Royal Prince Alfred Hospital and from the start I pumped the guys with the teachings of Vince Lombardi. One of Lombardi's messages to his men was: 'You will be successful if you are true to three things, and three things only: your family, your personal beliefs and the mighty Green Bay Packers.' Of course I modified his advice and drilled into my guys, 'Fellas, you will be successful against Queensland if you are true to three things, and three things only: your family, your personal beliefs and the New South Wales Blues.' Come match night, Origin I, and I was nervous, the team was nervous. The boys in their famous sky-blue jerseys were just about to run onto the field when I gathered them in a circle around me, looked each one solemnly in the eye and intoned, 'Fellas, you will be successful tonight if you are true to three things, and three things only: your family, your personal beliefs … *and the Green Bay Packers.*' What a start to our campaign – and things went south from there.

The team manager, Canterbury-Bankstown's Peter 'Bullfrog' Moore, and I tried to instil discipline. One of our hard-and-fast rules was that no New South Wales player was allowed to leave the camp without the permission of the coach and manager. The young Manly prop Phil Daley defied us. He later explained that he skipped camp because he had to attend to his business dealings and, as well, his wife was pregnant and he needed to see her, and he was afraid we wouldn't let him out. He was wrong.

If he'd approached us and explained his situation, we would have told him to do what he had to do, to go with our blessing, so long as he was back in time to train and play. But he didn't, and he left us with no alternative other than to sack him from the side. To do otherwise would have made a mockery of our discipline. Phil was devastated. It was a decision that Peter Moore, particularly, found hard to make because he was great mates with Phil's father, the Manly CEO Doug Daley.

State of Origin is very different to coaching a club side. Origin is a short campaign, spread over six weeks or so, and it is complicated further because the coach doesn't know many of his players terribly well. I had a few problems with Steve 'Blocker' Roach and in one match I had to pull him off the field because I felt he wasn't in form. He was furious with me. He forgave me, though, and in the off-season when Christine and I ran into Steve and his new wife, Cathy, at Club Med in Bali while they were on their honeymoon, we hung out together and were all great friends. I can't say that our newfound friendship extended to Blocker joining me on my runs around the island. He was definitely in relaxation mode.

Desperate Humour

Once again, in the wake of the State of Origin whitewash, I masked my despair with desperate humour. Nowadays, when I address gatherings I have a little routine about the thrashing we copped:

> Folks, for weeks after that Origin debacle, I was in such
> disgrace that I had to get around Sydney wearing dark glasses

and a false nose. I picked up the glasses cheap from my local chemist, and I'd like to now publicly thank Changa Langlands for the use of his schnoz in that dark period of my life.

After our loss in the first game, I decided the Blues had to go back to basics. I sat the boys down at training, held up a Steeden footy and began slowly, 'Now, men, take a good look. This is a football.' At that point, one of our front-rowers interrupted, 'Hang on, coach, you're going too fast.' Now, I have no intention of dobbing this bloke in – but his nickname is Blocker …

As had happened with Parramatta when I was replaced by Jack Gibson, Gibbo took over from me for Origin '89. Jack's team was beaten three–nil too.

Jack kept his job, though, and in 1990 brought me in as assistant coach. I reckon he wanted me there because I knew the names of his players. Jack was never great on names.

CHAPTER 12

Life After League

Last Tackle of the Set

Believe it or not, I had a life away from rugby league. I experienced the joys and heartbreaks of life, like everybody does. I loved my wife, Christine. We were soul mates and shared many interests, although, like all couples, we had a few ups and downs – always my fault and often to do with my partying ways and preoccupation with football.

I watched our daughters, Johanna and Amanda, grow up into beautiful and charming young women, being there for them through school and the trials of their teenage years.

My beautiful mother, Valda, rock of our family, fell to leukaemia in May, 1988. She was only sixty-nine years old. As anyone knows who has experienced it themselves or seen a loved one suffer, leukaemia is a terrible disease. Her diagnosis shattered us all but, typically, she got on with her life, fighting it with drugs and her great spirit. Until near the end, Mum still went to Bondi every morning to swim. I can still see her stroking through the water, and there on the beach with his rod is Dad.

With three mouths to feed I had always needed work outside rugby league. For some years I drove my concrete truck for Farley & Lewers at Botany; I worked as an advertising representative for Cumberland Newspapers while I was playing for the Eels during the late '70s. Then one day in 1978 I was walking past the Westfield shopping complex in Parramatta when I saw an abandoned shop. Until a week before it had been a struggling gift store, but now it was just an all-but-empty space with newspaper stuck all over the windows. For some reason I poked my head inside the door and I saw people packing items into tea-chests. I asked one fellow, 'Are you leaving?' And he told me he was, that their lease had expired and they had to move on. They were transferring all their stock to another store.

Suddenly I had a brainwave. I sought out the manager of Westfield Parramatta. 'My name's John Peard,' I told him. 'I want to open a sports store in that empty shop down there.'

So he sent me for an interview with one of the bosses at Westfield headquarters in William Street, between the city and Kings Cross. 'Have you had any experience in retail?' the Westfield bloke quite reasonably wanted to know.

'Nope,' I replied. 'But I know how to be nice to people and sell things, and I'm certain I could make a sports store a real goer. I know the sports gear manufacturers, and have a great relationship with Adidas.' (In reality, that great relationship with Adidas amounted to nothing more than the fact that I wore their boots.)

'Well,' he said, not sounding entirely convinced, 'we rarely take people on who have no experience, but we'll give it a go. Good luck, Mr Peard.' Then and there I signed a three-year deal with the management to open John Peard's Sports Store in Parramatta.

John Peard's Sports Store

I had the keys to what amounted to a room on the mall in the shopping centre: three walls, a door and a glass front. Everything else – shelves, counters, cash registers, stationery, sports gear to sell, staff to help me sell it, accountants, signage, advertising, building the business – was up to me.

Just when I was thinking I'd bitten off more than I could chew I bumped into an old footy friend, Garry Dowling, a dynamic fullback for Canterbury-Bankstown and Parramatta. (Not long after, he died in a terrible car smash.) Garry was a bit of a rogue who was always looking to make an easy buck. 'Listen, Bomber,' he said, 'I've got a bit of a sports store in Bankstown. There's some stock there. Why don't we combine forces. I'll whack my sporting goods into your store at Parramatta. I'll get more stock from the suppliers at the lowest wholesale prices because I've got a good credit rating. How's about you run the joint and we'll split the profits fifty-fifty?'

I shook hands with Garry. I was a sports store proprietor. I sold basic stock, nothing fancy. I did it on the cheap. Runners, tracksuits, some Parramatta Eels paraphernalia. Westfield required their tenants to pay for big, flash signs out the front to attract the customers, but I paid about two dollars for a polystyrene sign that read 'John Peard's Sports Store' and attached it to the shop's façade. People still came flocking.

Opening that store was one of the best things I ever did. Business boomed, as people rolled up to buy their equipment, chat to me about footy, maybe get an autograph. Soon I was making enough money to buy my business partner out and pay for my own stock from suppliers all over Sydney who knew they were on a winner with me. I put in new carpet and painted the place from top to bottom. We were doing really well.

Chris, Amanda and Johanna worked part-time for me, and really put in. Sometimes, too, I'd get the Eels players to come in and sell things, and the fanatical footy-loving fans of Parramatta jammed the joint wanting to meet and greet their local heroes. At semi-finals time, when footy fever really sweeps the district, Parramatta would be festooned with blue-and-gold streamers and bunting, and you literally couldn't move in my store as the public mobbed Artie, Sterlo, Brett Kenny, Mick Cronin, Peter Wynn, Bob O'Reilly and Ray Price. More than once there were so many Eels fans in the complex that store management had to switch the escalators off because they were scared that people would be hurt.

I employed four young blokes as sales assistants. Just like with my footballers, I talked to them about setting goals and being motivated. I'm happy to say that those guys went on to terrific business careers after getting a start with me.

After two years' slog, the sports store was going so well – retail turnover had increased by 40 per cent – that I felt confident in delegating responsibility to my staff. My friend Keiran Speed still reminds me that he was always bumping into

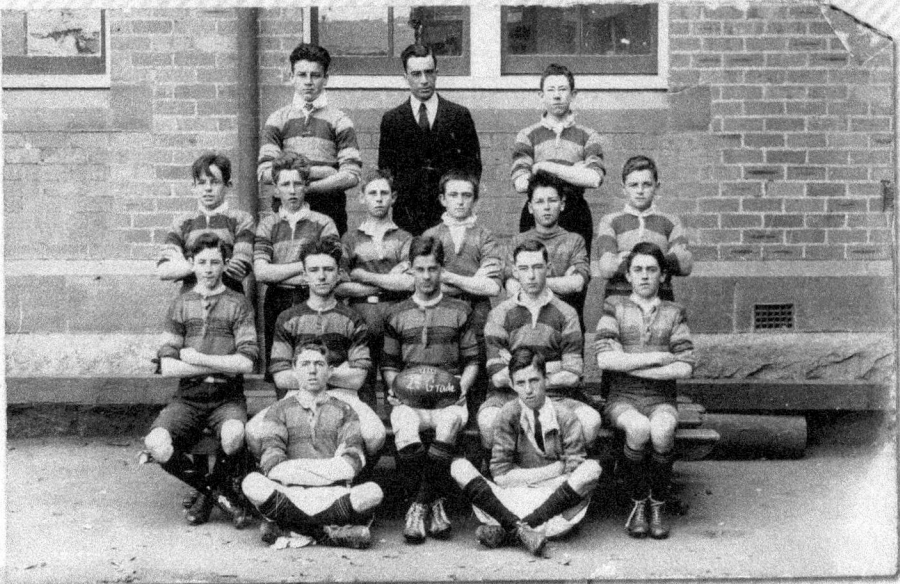

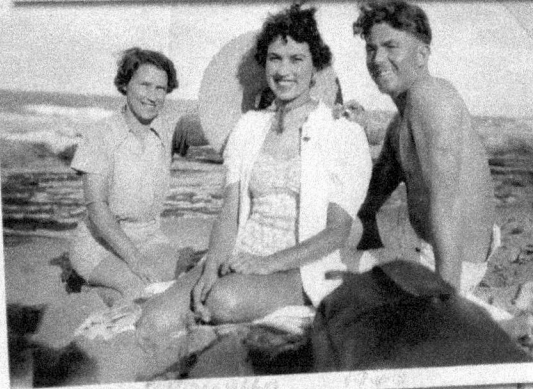

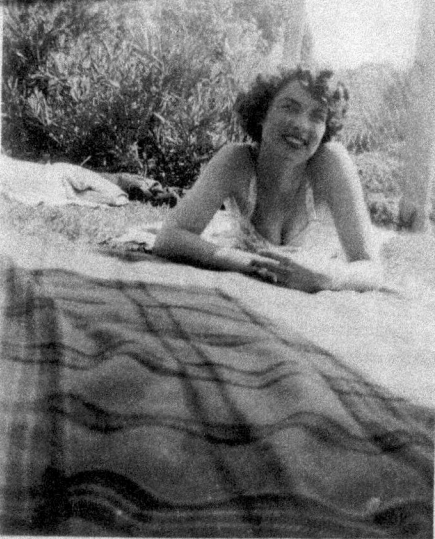

Images from a golden childhood

(*top*) That's my dad, Jack Peard, seated on the left at the front of his school rugby league team, in the early 1920s. Like me in my playing days, he was small, strong and quick; unlike me, however, he was a cheeky bugger on the field. I kept my head down and tried not to rev up opponents. (*middle*) Dad's great good fortune was meeting and falling in love with Valda, who became his wife and my mum. That's her in the centre, with an unknown friend (*at left*), in the early '40s. (*bottom*) Mum lived for her kids – even wearing my stiff new shoulder pads around the house to soften them up for me – but still found time to be a successful businesswoman and a loving wife to my dad.

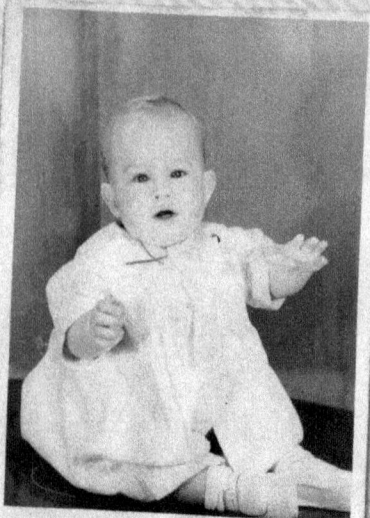

Believe it or not, I was good-looking once

… admittedly I was quite young *(above and above right)*. Here I am as a baby and toddler. Any good looks I was born with didn't last – thanks to the rigours of rugby league! *(below)* My doting dad and me, circa 1948. *(right)* 'A father of three! What happened?' Dad looks a little exasperated with *(from left)* me and my sisters Diane and Margaret during a day at the beach in the early 1950s.

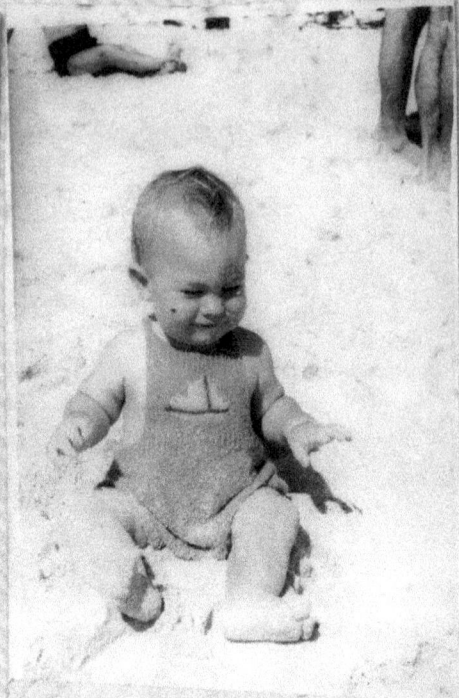

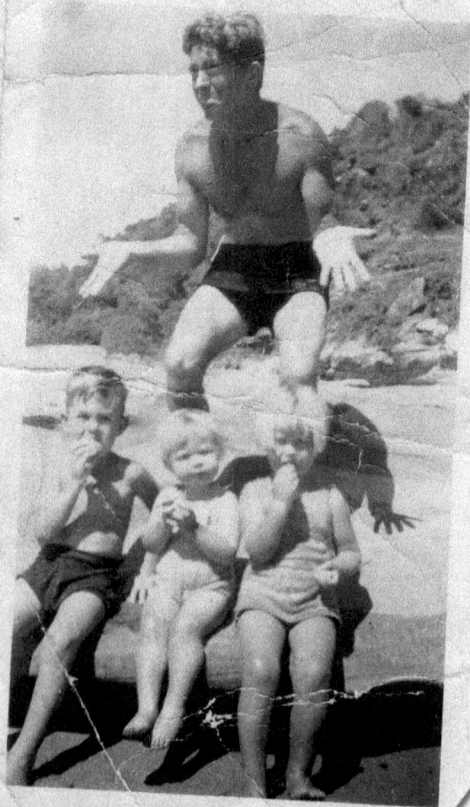

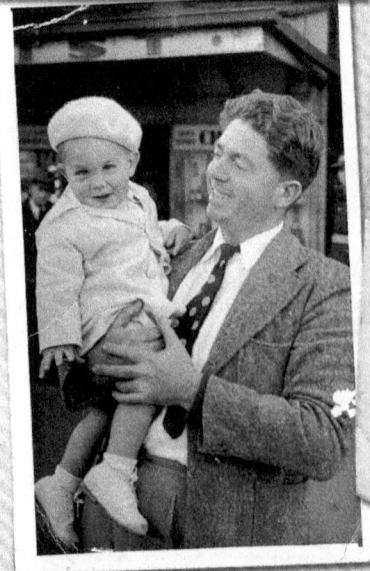

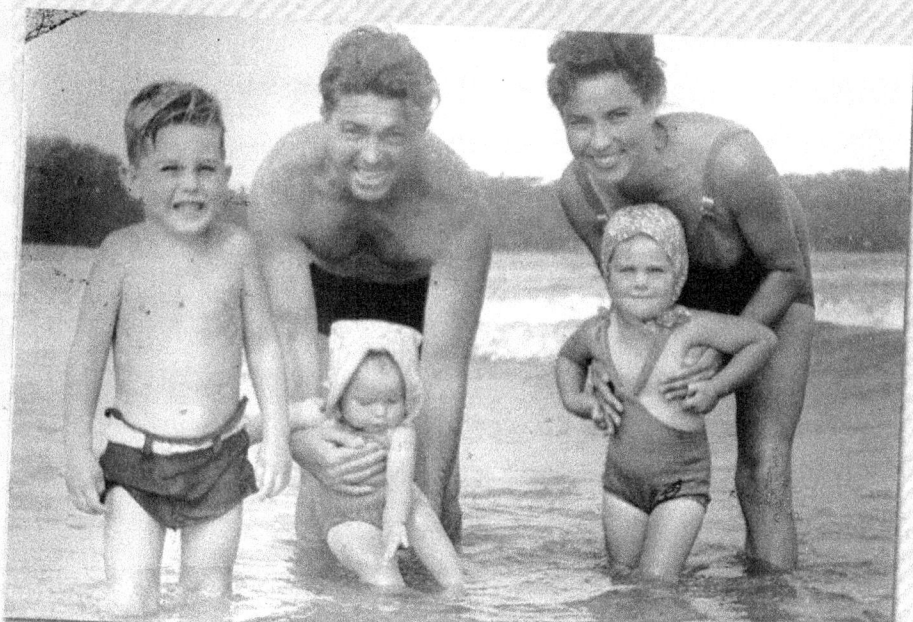

A water baby's progress

(*above*) Growing up, it seemed we were never out of the water. Here's me, Diane and Margaret at the beach with our parents. Mum's looking her most glamorous – no wonder Jack fell for her. (*below*) That's me on the far left in this photo of the Bondi junior R&R team. We won the Australian championship at Warrnambool in 1963. As in footy, I didn't let my diminutive size hamper me.

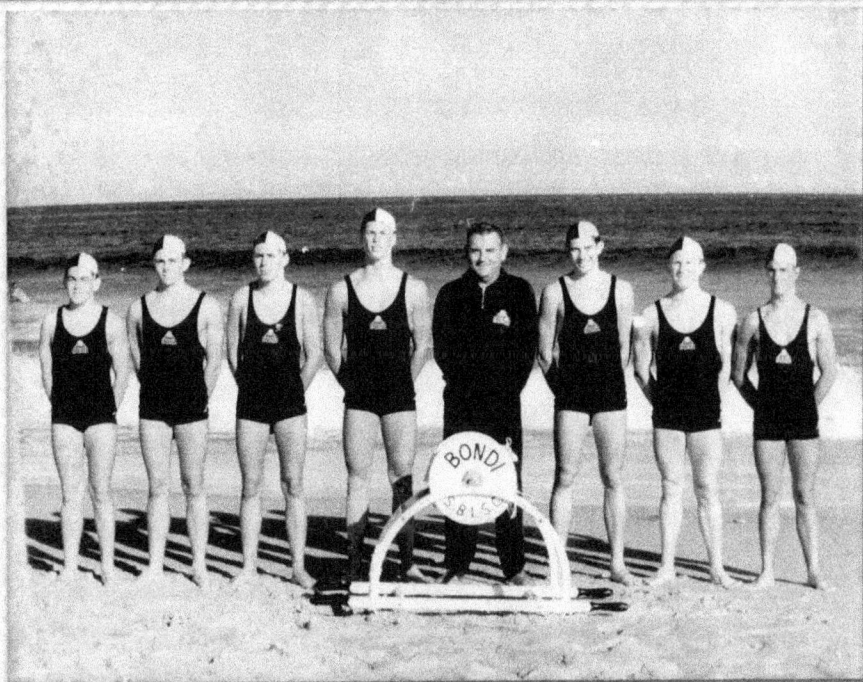

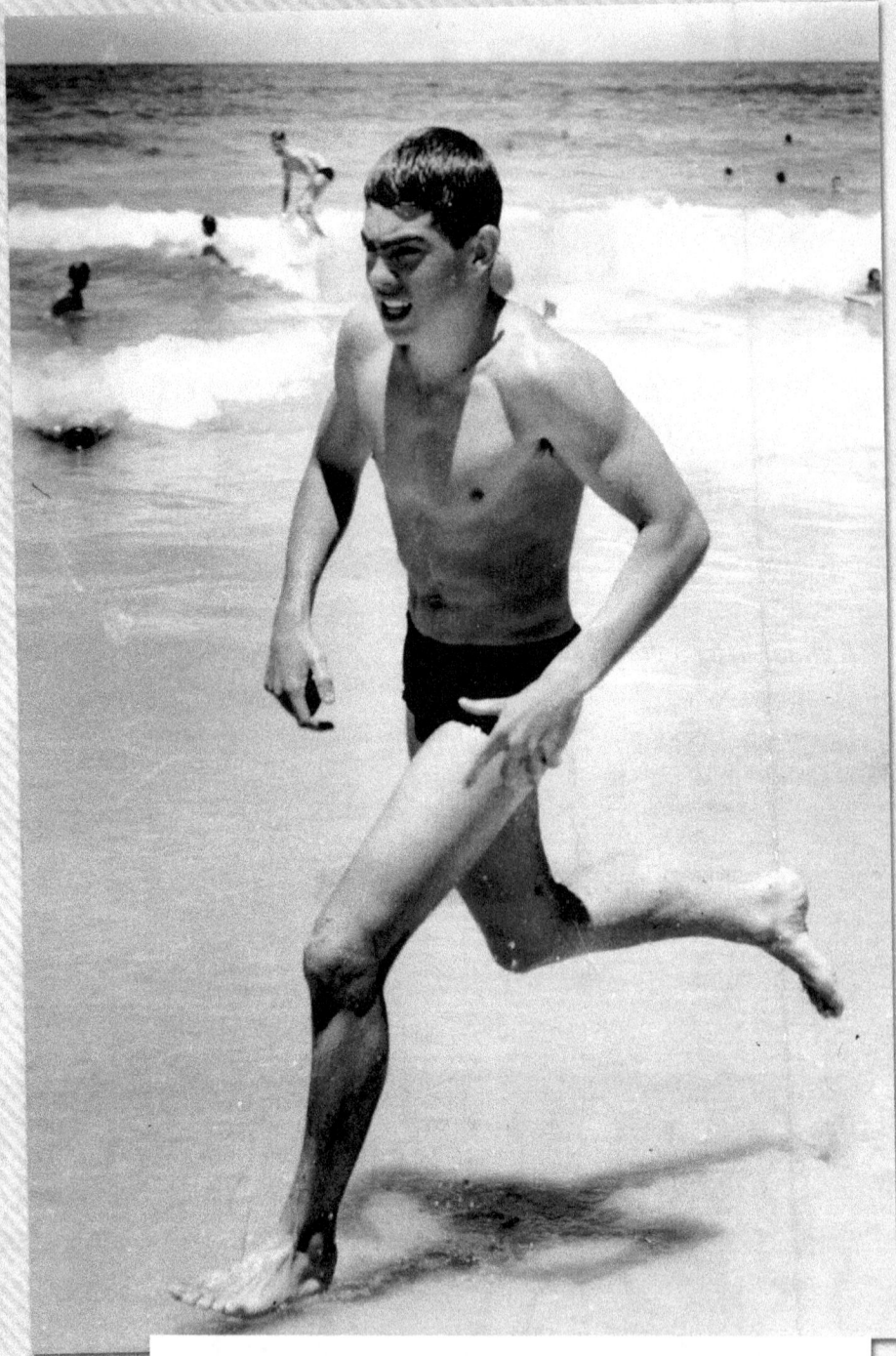

A life in the surf and sun

Through my teenage years, I surfed, played rugby league and
cricket, and ran … and ran. My playground was the eastern suburbs
of Sydney, blessed with beautiful beaches and parks. Naturally,
I accumulated many more sporting trophies than I did A grades.

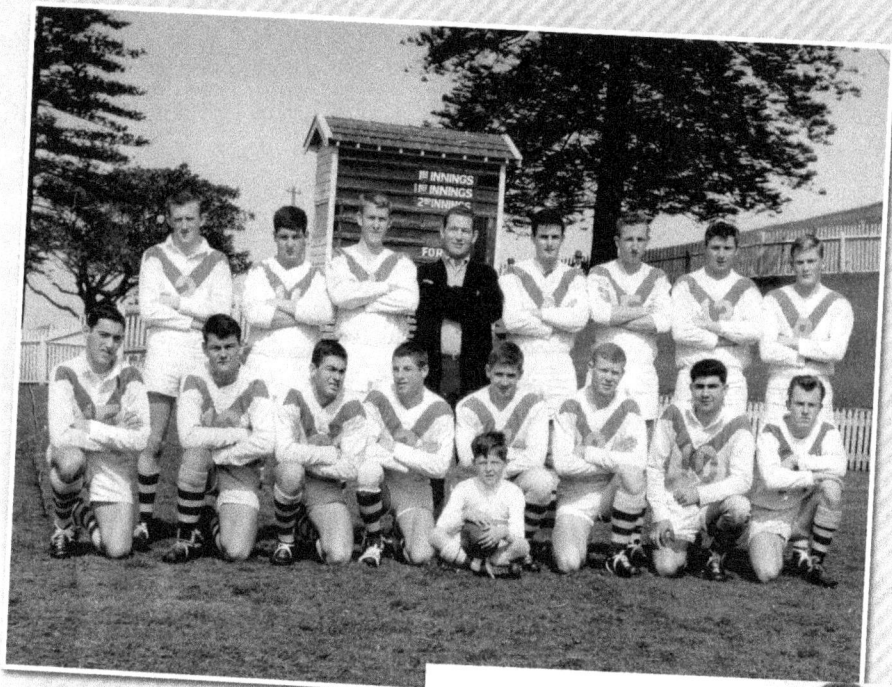

A rugby league career kicks off

(*above*) It was a natural step for me to move straight from my school league team to the local Bondi United junior side. I'm in the front row, third from the left, flanked by two guys who would be lifelong friends: John Shirley (*at left*) and Keiran Speed. We were a top team but always had our work cut out against the rougher Paddo Colts, whose star player and enforcer was my future Roosters' team-mate Bunny Reilly.

Family guy

(*right*) Domestic bliss: me at home in 1977 with my wife Chris and daughters Amanda and Johanna. There have been trials and tribulations in the years since, but today in 2007, in spite of everything, I'm proud to say we're still loving and close.

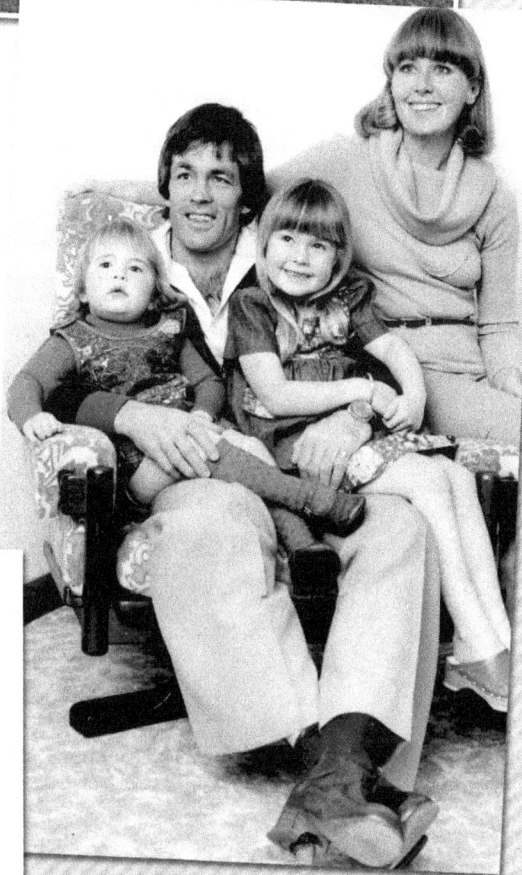

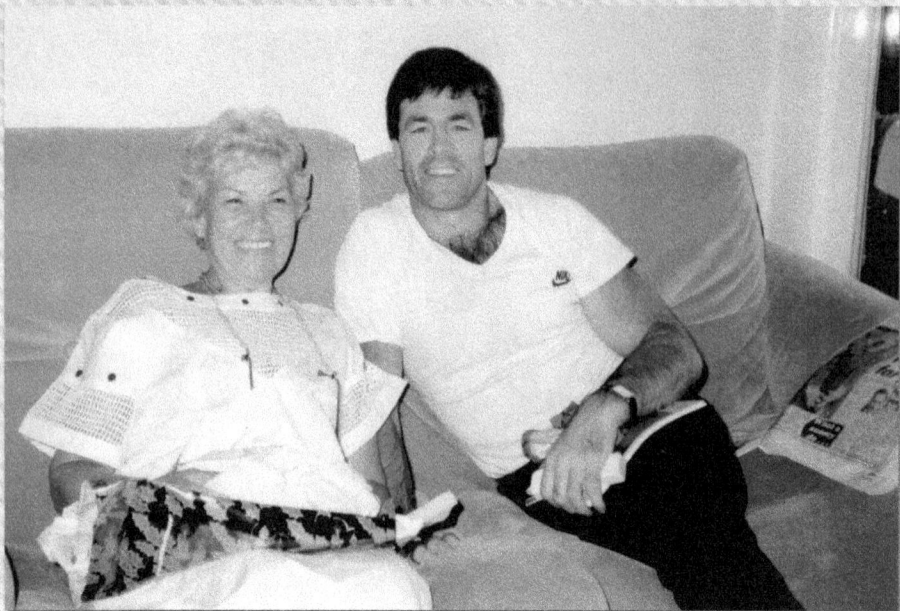

Into each life some rain must fall

(*above*) When this picture was taken, in the late '80s, Mum was dying of leukaemia. To the end, she was positive and in spite of the pain could always turn on that winning smile that won so many hearts during her lifetime. (*below*) After I had my stroke, it was my turn to smile through the pain. On the day this picture was taken, I took time off from rehab at Sutherland Hospital to enjoy a snack with well-wishers (*from left*) Chris, Bobby McMillan and his wife Rhonda, my daughter Amanda, Keiran Speed and my sister Diane, who'd come over from Western Australia.

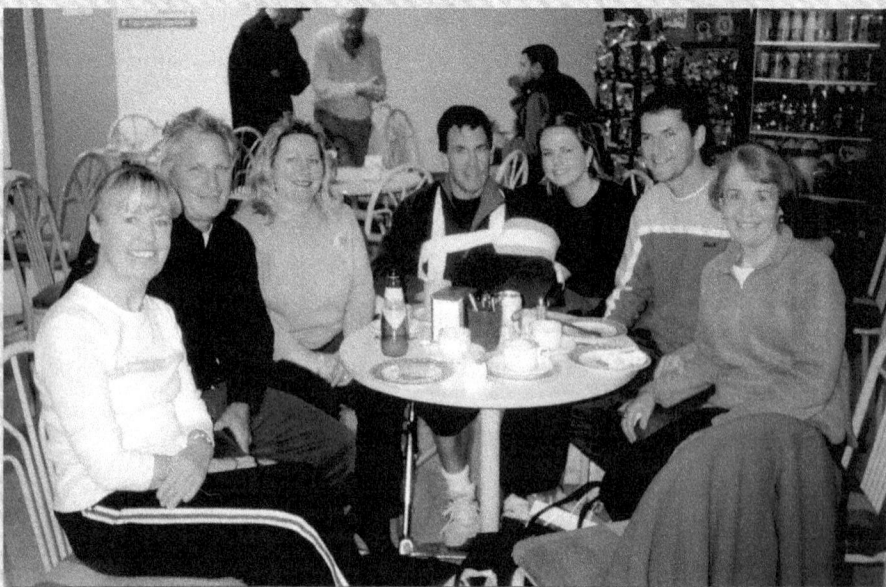

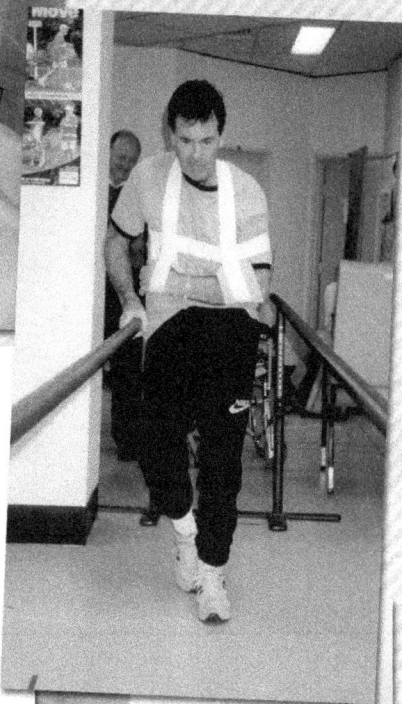

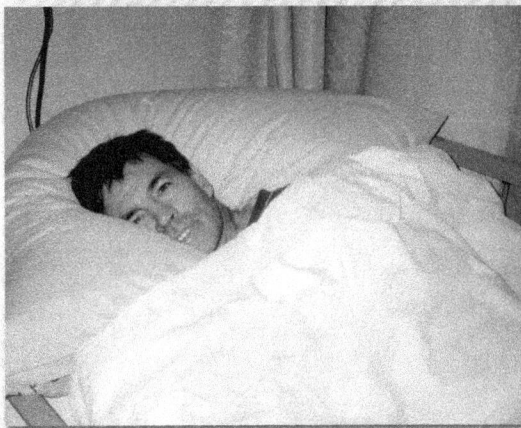

Stroke: my greatest challenge

(*above*) In the first days after I suffered my stroke on 6–7 June 2002, I lay immobile, lapsing in and out of consciousness. Some doctors said that I would be lucky to survive. (*right*) It was a pleasure to prove them wrong. As soon as I was physically able, I launched into my gruelling, sometimes heartbreaking, rehab therapy. There were tears and anger. Learning to function again became an obsession.

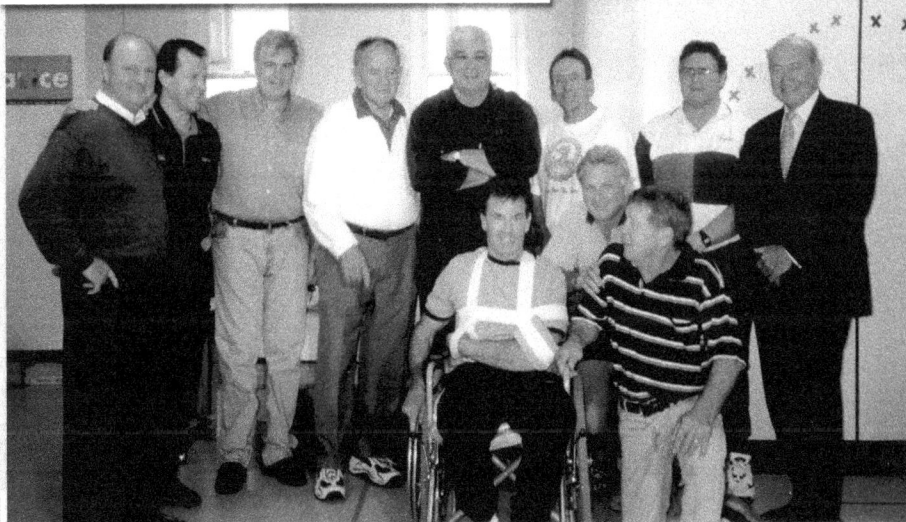

(*above*) The kindness of friends who called on me at the hospital to tell me to hurry up and get well was a great factor in my recovery. There's some serious footy talent among the bunch that came in this day: (*from left*) Royce Ayliffe, Graeme Hughes, Peter Cruikshank, Jack Gibson, Arthur Beetson, John Chisholm, unnamed (*sorry mate, I usually never forget a name*), John Quayle, and (*kneeling*) Bob McMillan and Billy Smith.

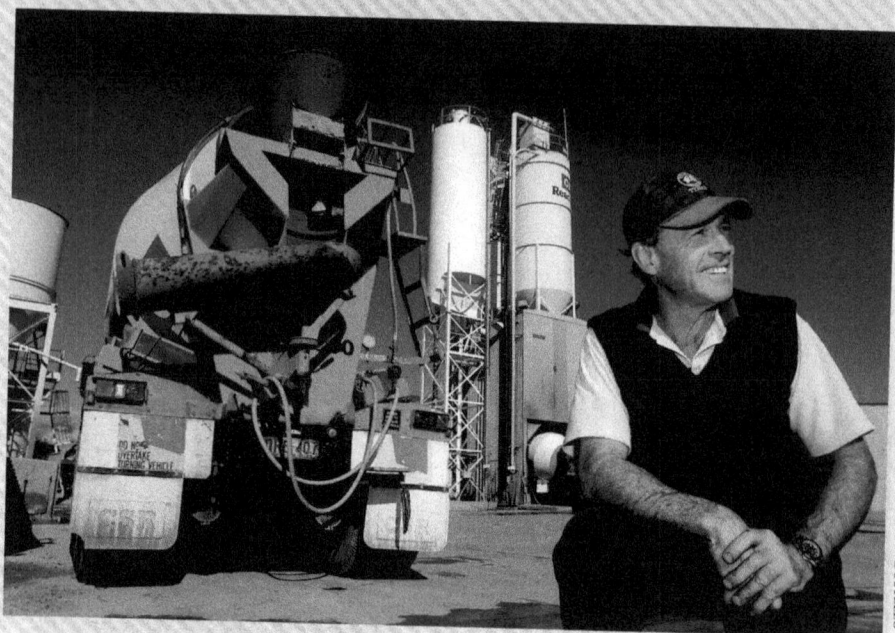

Newspix/News Ltd/Brett Costello

Pride and passion

(*above*) Until my stroke, I was a concrete contractor (*this is me with my truck in May 2002 just a few weeks before my stroke*), but now such physical work is impossible. Not that I'm idle. My days are filled with public speaking engagements all over Australia, visiting other stroke victims and enjoying myself with mates at the races and the rugby league. (*below*) My sister Margaret (centre, with Diane, our brother Geoff, Dad – not too long before he passed away – and me) says that since my stroke I've become more giving and loving. She's right. A brush with mortality sure helps you put life in perspective.

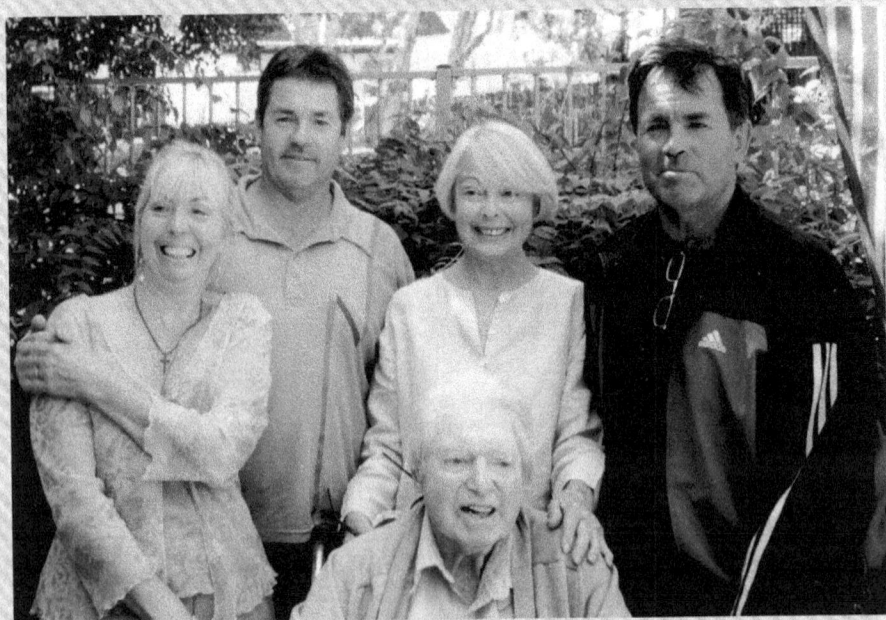

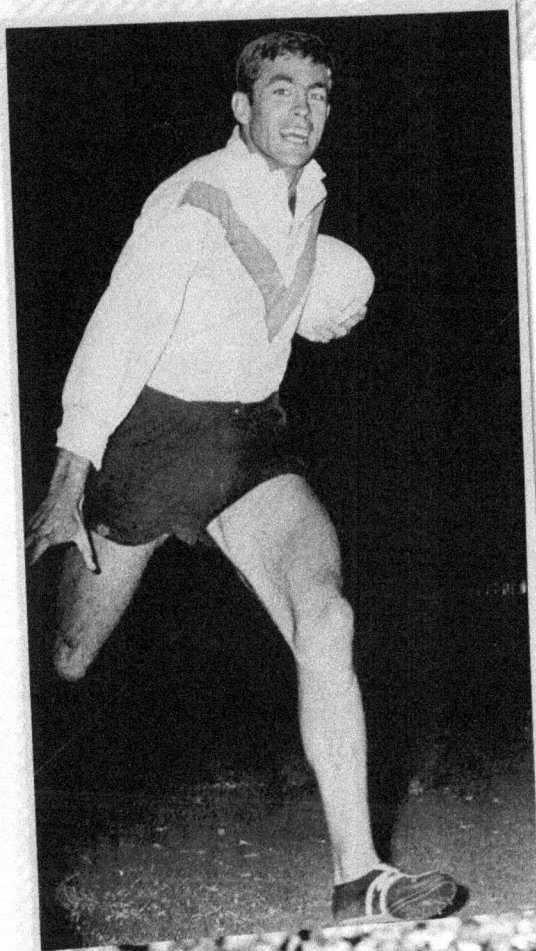

The greatest game

After earning my stripes at the Roosters from 1966 to '71 and at St George in 1972 and '73, I returned to Easts and experienced two golden years under coach Jack Gibson. Whether I was a young bloke (here at left, in my early grade days at the Roosters, and below getting collared by Balmain's Allan McMahon) copping a belting from better and bigger sides, or when winning premierships as a member of the crack Gibbo outfits of '74 and '75, I always loved my league – and it showed in the way I played the game.

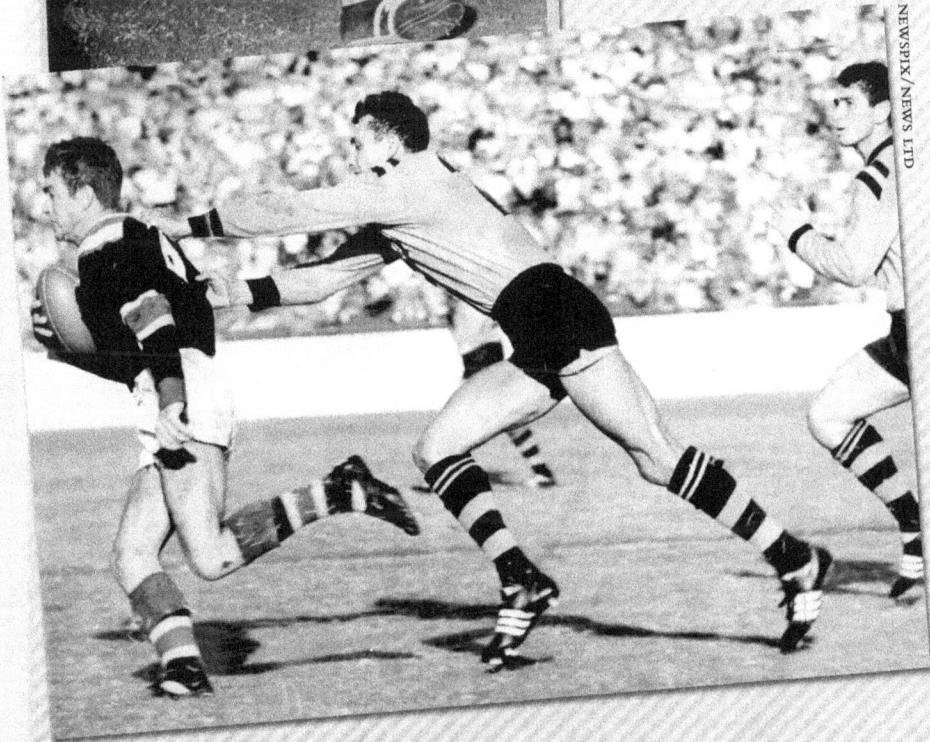

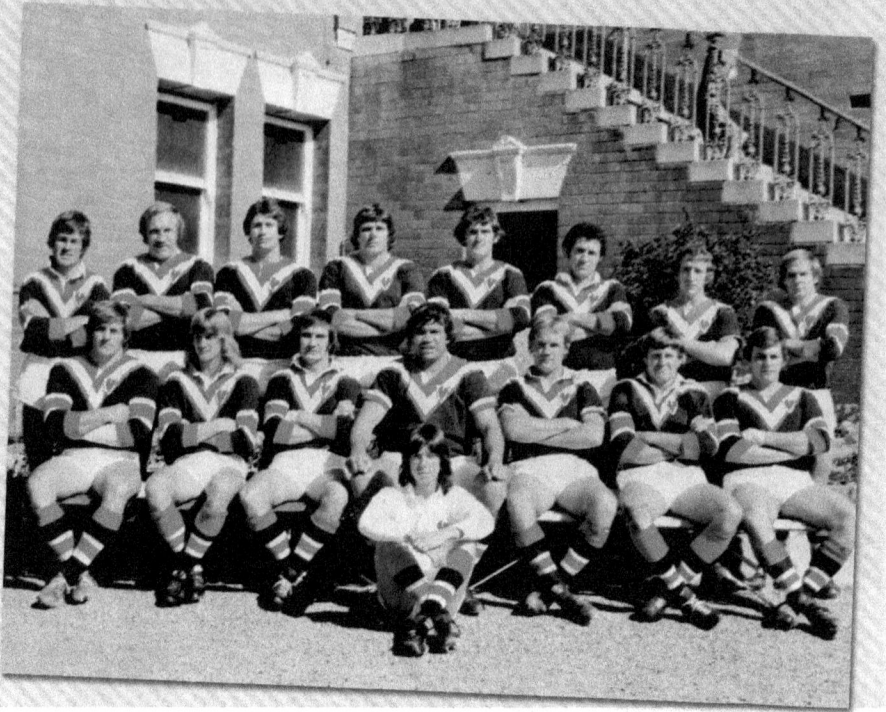

Glory days

(*above*) The premiership-winning Eastern Suburbs team of 1974, coached by Jack Gibson and captained by Arthur Beetson, has been called one of the finest club teams of all time. Back row, from left: yours truly, Mark Harris, Greg Bandiera, Laurie Freier, Bill Mullins, Jim Porter, Barry Reilly, Johnny Mayes; front row, from left: Elwyn Walters, Russell Fairfax, John Brass, Arthur Beetson, Ken Jones, Ron Coote, Ian Mackay. (*below*) Scoring a try. I must have been returning from injury because I'm wearing number 44.

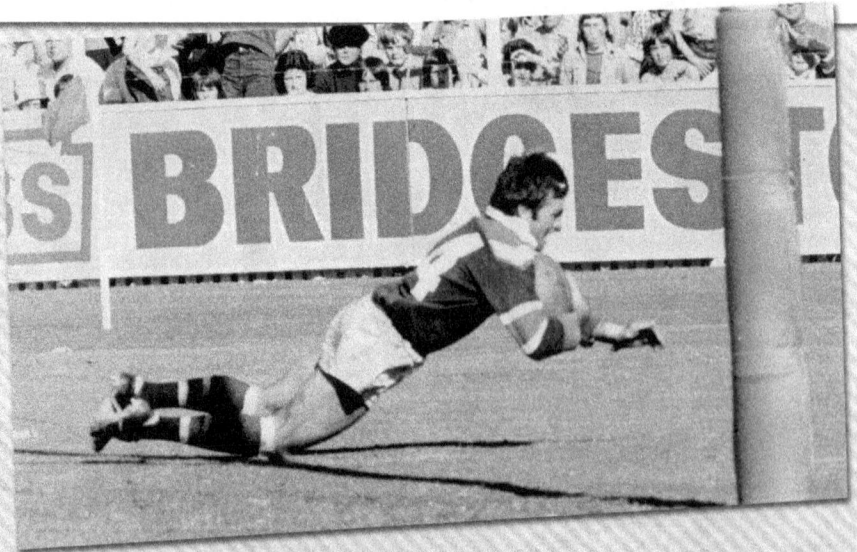

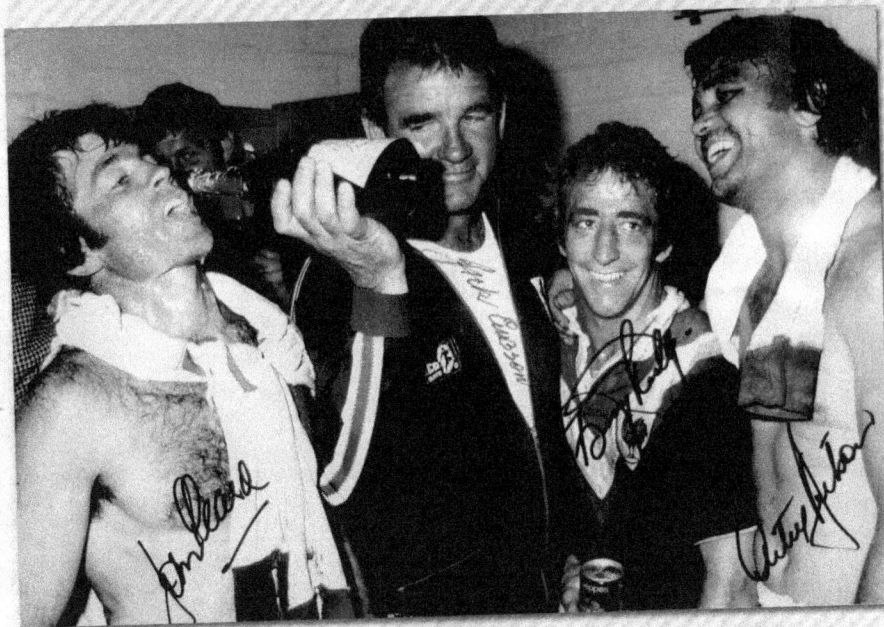

NEWSPIX/NEWS LTD

Champagne style

(*above*) After we walloped
Canterbury-Bankstown 19–4 in
the 1974 grand final, Jack Gibson,
Bunny (Barry) Reilly, Artie Beetson
and I let down our hair in the
dressing room. Jack cracked an
uncharacteristic smile as he cracked
the champers. Didn't last. Before
long we were back in training for
our successful 1975 title defence.
(*right*) Easts fullback Russell Fairfax
(number 1) leaps high to pluck one
of my bombs out of the air.
Ironically, the bloke to Russell's
left so fiercely contesting the ball
is Parramatta's Ray Price, who
would become the beneficiary of
my high punts when I shifted to
Parra in 1976. Both players chased
down my bombs like rabid
terriers, and woe betide anyone
who got in their way.

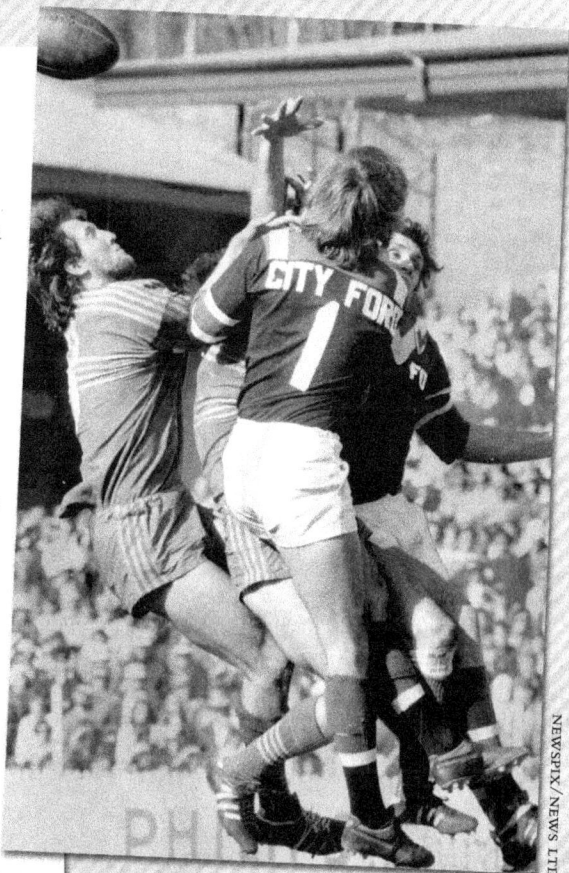

NEWSPIX/NEWS LTD

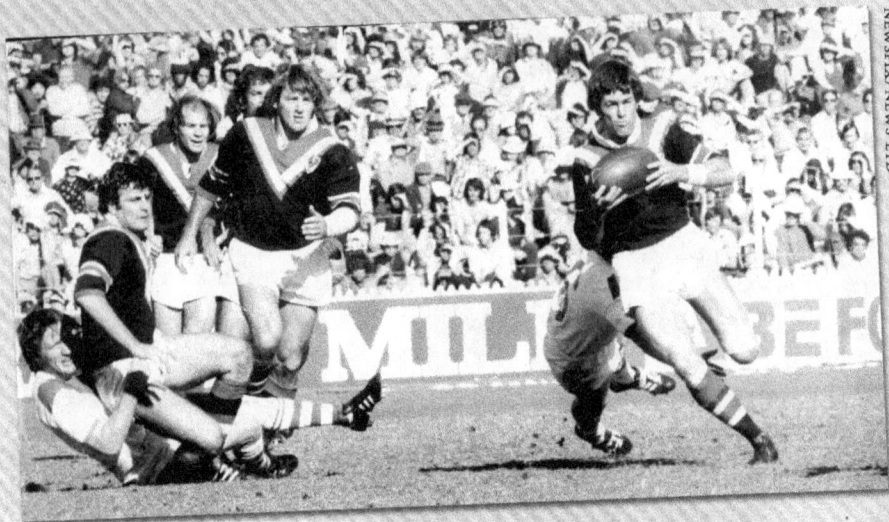

Centre stage

(*above*) Although I was known as a steady, hard-tackling team player with a good passing and kicking game, I was faster and more elusive than I looked, and often, as in this 1975 semi-final match at the SCG, against St George, found myself in the clear with the ball. (*right*) It was no fluke that my game improved out of sight after I linked up with Jack Gibson and Arthur Beetson at the Roosters in 1974 and '75. I went from being a sound club player to an international representing my country in Tests against New Zealand, Wales, England and Great Britain and my state against Queensland.

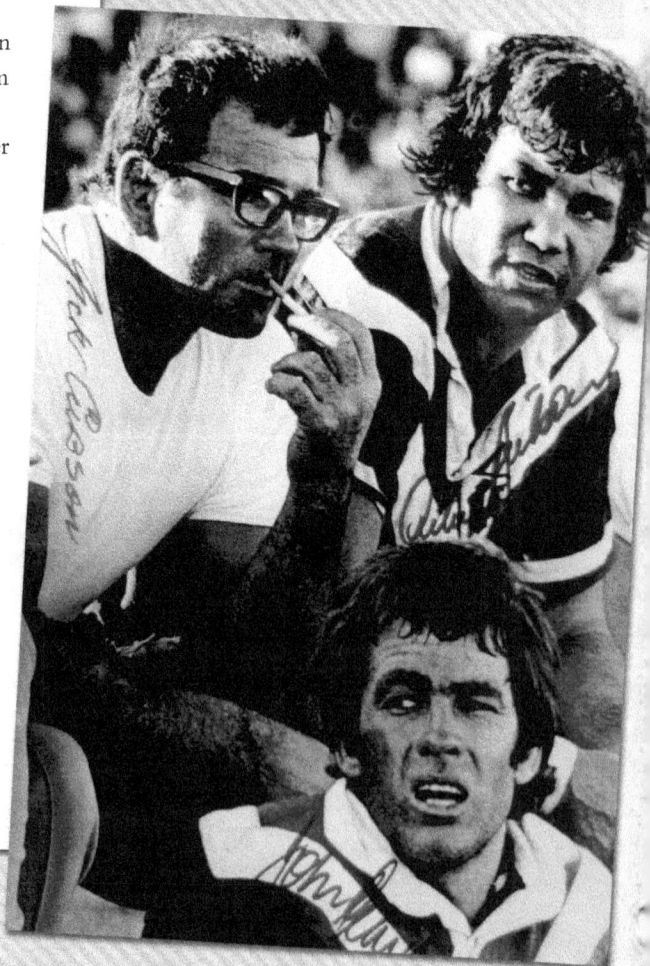

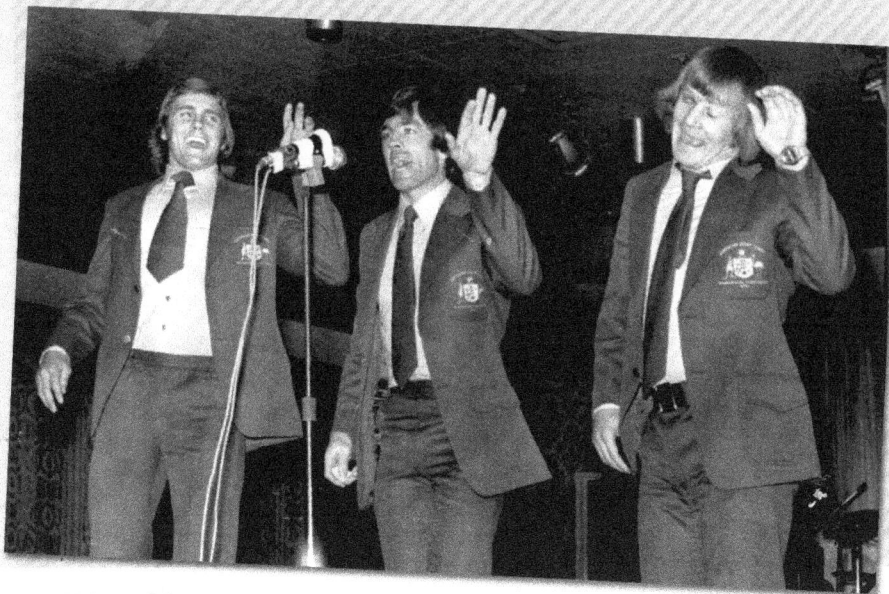

Larrikins at large

(*above*) On tour with the Australian World Series team in November 1975, Greg Pierce (*left*), Tommy Raudonikis and I put on an impromptu show for the crowd at Salford club's Rugby League Gala Night. Fortunately, I kept no reviews! In recent years both Greg and Tommy, so indomitable in their playing days, have bravely battled illness.

The hard yards

(*below left*) There was no secret to my accurate kicking. I practised endlessly, both at training (here in June 1976) and in my own time, booting a succession of balls into the air and landing them exactly where I wanted them. (*below*) Ever since I was a boy playing backyard footy I got a kick out of tackling. My love of smashing a bigger bloke continued throughout my career. Here I'm grassing the rampaging Manly and Australian fullback Graham Eadie during the 1976 grand final.

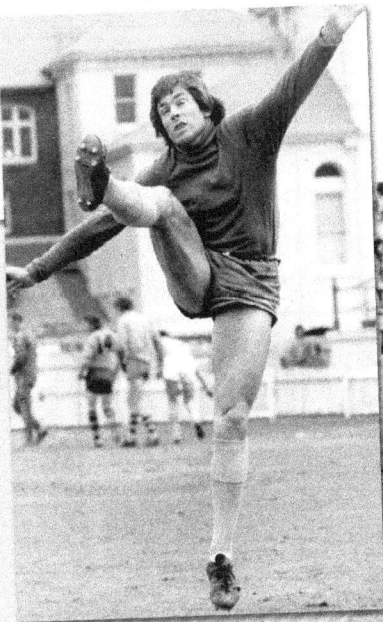

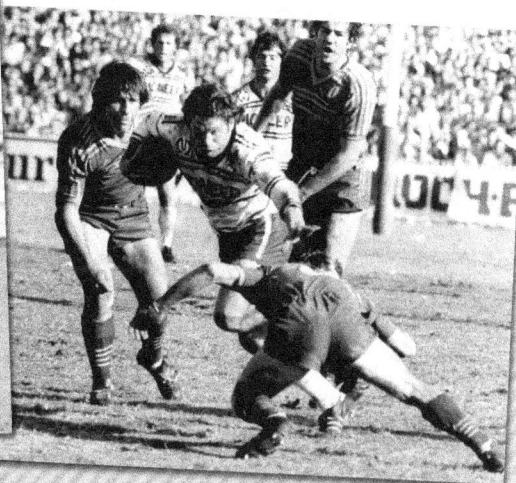

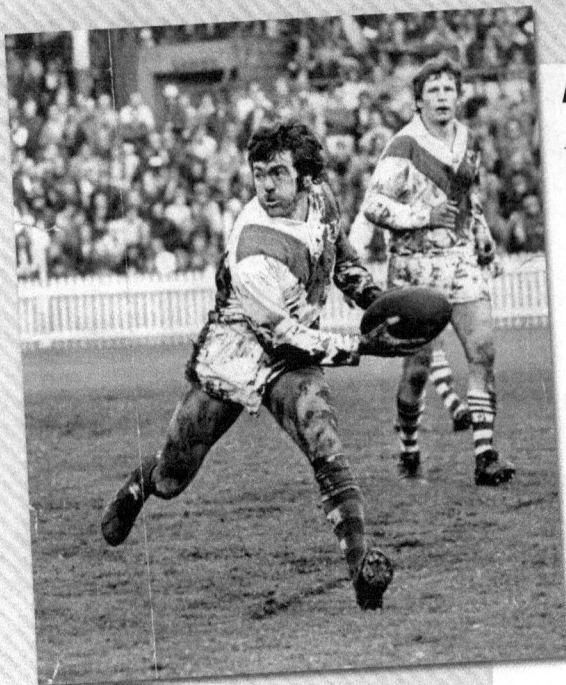

Fundamentally sound ...

As a kid I learned the basic skills of rugby league thoroughly. I figured that if you passed, kicked and tackled in textbook fashion, and could combine these fundamentals with guts, fitness and stamina, and the ability to use your brain, you'd do OK in our brutal and unforgiving code. Here, during my St George days, I'm running with the ball held out in front of me, just as all my coaches taught me, ready to pass to a support or wrong-foot the defence and dash through the gap myself. Backing up is sturdy Saints forward Graeme Sams.

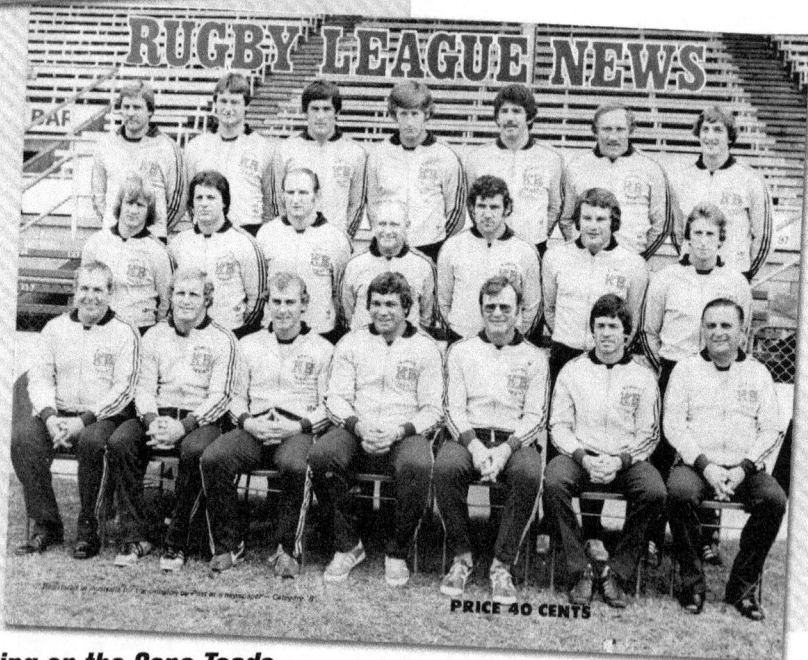

Taking on the Cane Toads

My Parramatta coach Terry Fearnley (*front row, third from right*) coached New South Wales in 1977, and I joined my Parramatta team-mates Denis Fitzgerald (*back row, fourth from left*), Graham Olling (*second row, third from left*), Mick Cronin (*second row, fifth from left*) and Ray Higgs (*front row, second from left*) in the blue jumper. My old Roosters team-mates Mark Harris and Artie Beetson were in the side too.

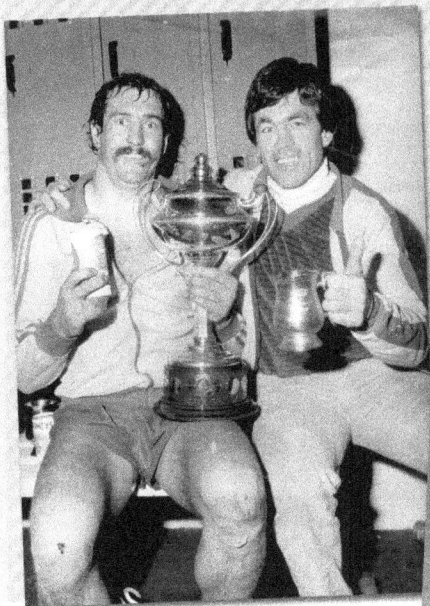

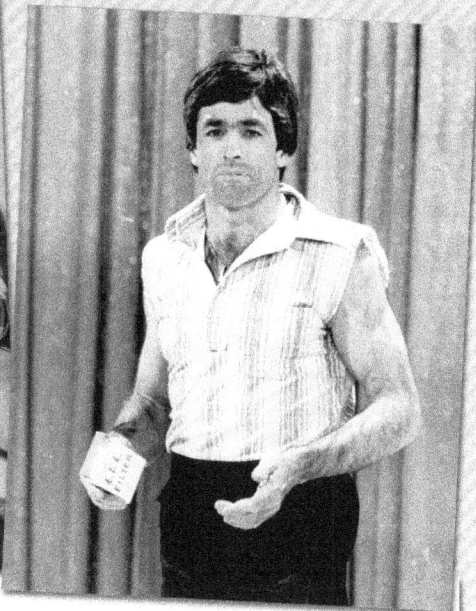

Coach and comedian

(*above left*) I won no premierships coaching Parramatta and Penrith, but in 1978 my Parramatta Eels did win the lucrative Tooth Cup midweek competition. Helping me celebrate with the sponsor's product is the tough and huge-hearted Ron Hilditch. (*above right*) My comedy act today has evolved from my early attempts at impersonating Paul Hogan.

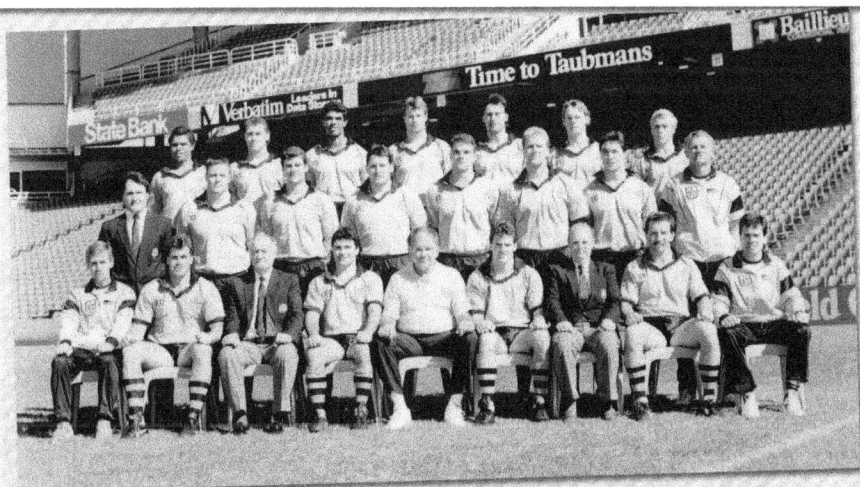

Among the giants

(*above*) In 1990, Jack Gibson was appointed coach of the New South Wales State of Origin side, and when he asked me to be his assistant I leapt at the chance. The side featured some of the greatest players our game has seen in Ricky Stuart, Andrew Ettingshausen, Glenn Lazarus, Steve Roach, Ian Roberts, Paul Sironen, Bradley Clyde, David Gillespie, Ben Elias and Michael O'Connor. It was a pleasure to be involved.

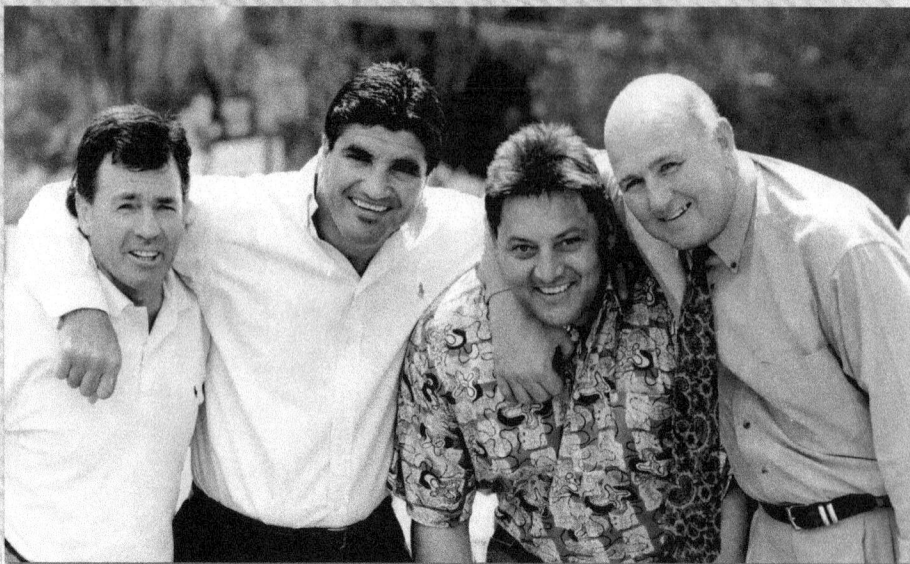

TWEED NEWSPAPER CO (DAILY NEWS)

Brotherhood of champions

Rugby league players give each other no quarter on the field, but off it, I'm glad to say, there's a bond that often lasts a lifetime between the men who play this take-no-prisoners sport. The wonderful Men of League organisation that looks after old players having tough times is typical. (*above*) Here, Mario Fenech, Steve Roach and yours truly, along with an acquaintance who joined us for the photo, catch up circa 2000. And (*below*) the mighty Artie Beetson, Graeme Langlands and Johnny Raper and I still cross paths many times a year at rugby league functions. Long may it last.

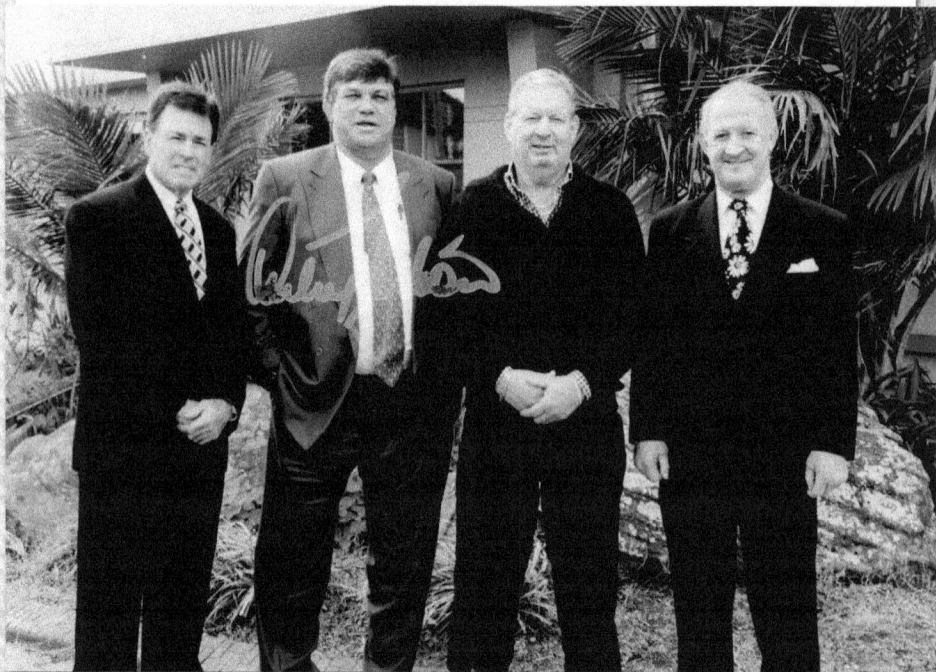

me at the Sydney Football Stadium playing tennis with John Quayle or swimming or lifting weights in the gym and when he'd ask me why I wasn't at work, I'd tell him, 'Oh, no worries, Speedy, someone's minding the store.'

With business booming at Parramatta I opened another shop, in Liverpool. In due course, I sold Liverpool to John Young, the kid from next door in Blakehurst all those years before, who came to the park with me to catch my bombs.

But by 1993, with rising costs, making good money out of the business was getting harder. I decided to sell up and find new challenges.

Football was in my heart still, and I'd taken a position as assistant coach at the Roosters in 1992, working mainly with the younger players and doing a bit of talent-scouting, which took me to the bush, a place this city boy had come to love.

The motivation bug had really bitten me deep. I was applying the teachings of Vince Lombardi, Jack Gibson and other inspiring motivators to all areas of my life – to footy, to work, to day-to-day doings with my family. Strive hard to reach your potential; set goals and work to achieve them. I bought books and tapes, enough to fill entire boxes at my home. I read those books devotedly, and listened to the tapes in my car as I trekked from Cronulla to Parramatta. Did I take it all too seriously? Probably, but that didn't invalidate the truth that prosperity and happiness were there for the taking if you did your very best.

A Double Act with Artie

I'd always fancied myself as a bit of a comedian. I had the happy knack of making people laugh. So when I overdosed on the taped messages of the motivators on those tedious trips to and from the Sutherland Shire, I'd pop a comedy tape into the car player to give me a laugh. Bill Cosby, Brian Doyle, Kevin 'Bloody' Wilson, Danny McMaster, Ray Seagar, Hal Roach, Col Reilly, Johnny Garfield and Paul Hogan really broke me up, and sometimes I nearly ran off the road I'd be laughing so much. Almost without realising it I learned how these blokes constructed a joke or a hilarious yarn. How they'd elaborately set up the punchline and then deliver it perfectly for maximum comic effect.

I wondered whether I could create jokes, making light of things that I knew about and were close to my heart: rugby league, horseracing, drinking and betting, the knockabout idiosyncrasies of family and friends. Whenever an opportunity arose I'd tell these jokes, my own and ones I'd pinched from others, to friends and at football gatherings, and people would fall about laughing, just as I did when listening to my comedian heroes. More than once the thought occurred to me on those long drives that if ever worse came to worst, I could stand up in front of a crowd and pay the bills by making people laugh.

The ABC, of all people, gave me a chance to test out my material when in 1992 they offered me the job of being a co-commentator alongside Arthur Beetson and David 'Thirsty' Morrow, and later Warren Boland, on their Saturday rugby league TV broadcasts, after my coaching stint at Parramatta came to an end. I was very much the low man on the totem pole, expected to provide colour, dry Aussie humour and the occasional insight from my vantage point on the sideline; maybe bring up something I'd seen that neither Artie, Thirsty nor Warren had mentioned. Arthur and I merely kept up the banter we had shared from our years at the Roosters and the Eels. I was always having a go at Arthur about his weight. Once, after the referee had allowed a dodgy try, Arthur commented on air, 'Bomber, if that was a try, I'll walk home!'

I shot straight back: 'You'll be sweet, Artie, it's a six-lane highway.'

We were on the same wavelength and listeners, judging by the feedback the ABC received, enjoyed our double act.

In those days, there was an open microphone so I was able to butt in whenever I liked, and not wait for a signal from the producer inviting you to comment, which is what happens with football calls today. And unlike talkback radio, there was no five-second delay on our footy calls, so bloopers, embarrassing mistakes and off-colour jokes made it to air.

One day we were at North Sydney Oval and Arthur said, 'Jeez, that Norths forward Josh Stuart is a tough kid ...' and I piped up, 'He sure is, Arthur, he's tougher than a Jewish landlord.' The switchboard came to life. It glowed, rattled and hummed and looked like it was about to explode. Seems a few thousand people out there in radio land had taken exception to my quip.

The producer rushed over to me at the end of the match. 'John,' he said, with terror in his eyes, 'you're going to have to apologise on air for what you said.'

So I did. And I thought while I was at it, I may as well try, as my motivational mentors had taught me, to turn a negative into a positive and flog a bit of sports gear. In the most contrite voice I could muster I said, 'Listeners, I'm sorry if I've offended. I've nothing against Jews. In fact, I used to live in Rose Bay ... and some of my very best customers at my sports stores at

Parramatta and Liverpool are Jewish.' The switchboard lit up all over again.

'Can You Hear a Crackling Noise?'

Quite often after calling the day's game, I'd then interview one of the players – not necessarily the man of the match, just someone who could speak a bit. Maybe a garrulous rogue like Johnny Elias. Once, at Newcastle, after completing my usual post-match interview, I disconnected the cord from my headphones and raced to the car park, eager to get into my beaten-up old station wagon and drive off down the highway to Sydney.

On the way, I noticed people were looking at me intently, but figured they recognised me from my football days or had seen me on ABC footy broadcasts on TV. I smiled and waved graciously.

By Swansea, just south of Newcastle, I was a little thirsty. In those pre–random breath-test days, I was among that legion of drivers who (incredibly, in hindsight today) thought nothing of sipping from a can of beer while driving. So I stopped at a bottle shop and said to the young bloke behind the counter, 'Four cans of Tooheys, mate. That should get me home.'

The fellow went to the cold room and returned with the beers and bagged them. As I paid him, I asked, 'Can you hear a crackling noise?'

'No,' he said.

'I can. It sounds like waves breaking on the seashore.'

'I can't hear a thing.'

'Are you positive you can't hear a crackling noise?' I asked again.

He said, 'Mate, it wouldn't be those earphones you've got on, would it?'

'Oh shit …' How stupid did I feel! I'd pulled the cord from my broadcasting headphones but left the bloody ear-cans on.

I realised then that those people staring at me from their cars weren't thinking, 'What a star!' They were thinking, 'What a dickhead, wearing his headphones in the car. He thinks he's bloody Sir Charles Kingsford Smith!'

Peter Jackson

Arthur moved on to new pastures and he was replaced on the ABC Saturday broadcasts by the charismatic larrikin Peter Jackson. Peter was as good at making people laugh as he had been at playing football for Canberra, Norths, Queensland and Australia. Later, after Peter committed suicide in November 1997, we all found out that he suffered from depression. He was always such fun that it never occurred to me that deep down inside he was struggling desperately against demons that would soon overwhelm even his great spirit. The only thing I noticed was that Jacko was occasionally edgy and anxious and a little fidgety. Peter's death was a loss to all who knew him.

I soldiered on behind the microphone until the end of the 1993 season – having had great times with Thirsty, Morrow and Jacko.

Footy in the Bush

Today, when Arthur and I go to the bush to speak and promote rugby league, people come up to us and ask why the ABC stopped broadcasting that Saturday afternoon game, which was beamed out to all of Australia. Watching it was a much-anticipated weekly highlight for many thousands of far-flung people who had no hope of seeing the big games live and who gathered in the pub or around their fire at home on a cold arvo to see the best players in the world and hear the commentary. I know I speak for Arthur Beetson too when I say that it's a shame it's a thing of the past. Rugby league lost heavily, too.

I fear that our game is dying in its heartland, the bush. And this is not just doom and gloom from a city slicker. I've travelled extensively through rural New South Wales and Queensland on my speaking engagements and I've seen what's happening first hand. The message I get everywhere I go is that the game is struggling, and that many of the schools out there that always played league don't play it any more. Soccer, Aussie Rules and rugby union are making a play for the hearts and minds of the kids. Many of the senior league teams have died and the ones that have survived face a never-ending struggle to raise money.

We have to revive the game in the country by sending NRL players to the bush on PR duty. It's all very well to have a successful NRL comp with its big-city following and mega-buck TV deals, but if the grassroots wither, where will the stars of the future come from?

I also have an issue with the NRL clubs snatching promising country players as young as fifteen and sixteen. Never can they say, 'I played first grade for my home town.' Look at the Country team that plays City each year. There's not a single player in the side that doesn't play for an NRL club. Another solution may be to assign each NRL club a bush region, and make the Roosters or the Tigers or the Eels responsible for the welfare of their country cousin's football. Players from the bush could be drafted into the senior team.

My Best Mate

In 1993, an eventful year for me, Christine and I split up after twenty-four years of marriage. I take full responsibility. I made mistakes and did dumb things. I admit I was selfish. I and my loved ones were victims of my need to party hard, as well as the self-centredness I'd been prone to since childhood. Too often I put myself first.

Happily, Christine and I never stopped being friends, not even in the dark days when we separated, and today she remains one of my best mates. No one was kinder to me when I had my stroke than Chris. I'll love her till the day I die.

Work Hard and Play Harder

To survive the great upheaval in my life I kept myself busy, but in quiet moments I knew that I had made one of the worst blunders a man can make.

The '90s seemed to flash by so fast and before long a new millennium was looming. I became popular on the public-speaking circuit, and spent a few days each month travelling to various clubs throughout New South Wales and Queensland. I worked for a time as a bookmaker's clerk, often at terrific country racetracks such as Coffs Harbour and Grafton. Then I bought another concrete truck. I knew that business, and that if I worked hard it could provide me with a good living. As an owner-driver, it's your truck, it's their barrel of concrete. You have to look after both, clean them and grease them and all that, but you're paid reasonable rates. You can make $110,000 a year gross. Then, of course, you have to pay your costs, your tyres, your fuel.

I relished the stresses of having to deliver my load on time in spite of the worsening Sydney traffic. At the work site I'd dump my load and then, even though I didn't have to, I'd grab a spare wheelbarrow and wheel the wet concrete to the job. A barrow-ful of concrete is not light. It can weigh ninety kilos or more.

To relax after back-breaking, muscle-straining days, I went to the football and to the races. To pubs and clubs. I partied hard and drank probably more than was good for me. I had a thousand friends. 'Work hard and play harder' was my motto, and my life.

It was in the early '90s that lifting weights, which I had always done as a means to an end – that is, to be a better sportsman – became an end in itself. I worked out with them every day and before long it was nothing for me to throw 100-kilo barbells around like corks.

I often trained at a gym called the Century Health Studio at Condell Park, where Graham Olling and Ray Price worked out when we were at Parramatta. The old bloke who ran the joint, George Chappell, could lift three times his own body weight. He was an inspiration. I'd also been inspired by the feats of Australian weightlifter Dean Lukin, who won a gold medal at the 1984 Olympic Games. He had to clean and jerk 240 kilos to win it.

I became interested in the power clean, in which you pull the bar up to your clavicle and use your body as a fulcrum to lift the weight. I obviously couldn't get anywhere near 240 kilos, but I could handle well over 100 kilos, which was pretty good for a bloke over fifty. I went to either the gym at Condell Park or the one at North Cronulla surf club every single afternoon – that's how into lifting I was.

CHAPTER 13

A Funny Thing Happened ...

A Talent to Talk

My sister Margaret was one of the first to believe that I could stand up and entertain an audience. She tells the story of the time in 1991 when she invited me to a gala dinner to celebrate the centenary of Rose Bay Public School, where she was headmistress and which we'd all attended as kids.

'They were a very mixed group of parents at the school,' She begins. 'We had Russians, we had lots of Jewish people and we had quite a few Chinese folk. Aussies and Brits of course, some South Africans.

'I asked John to say a few words after dinner. Not because I had any idea that he could speak in public, but because he'd gone to the school and had been a prominent sportsman.

'I had this fabulous teacher on my staff, named Peter Tomlin. Peter was a very good speaker, and he offered to MC the event. Well, Peter was having a terrible time because none of the parents wanted to listen to him. They kept talking to each other right over the top of him. The night was turning into a disaster. Peter, who was usually a master at crowd control, was getting irritated and saying things like, "You people over there! Please stop talking, I'm trying to announce the proceedings …"

'I was worried for John. How on earth would he be able to make his speech with this rowdy bunch talking over the top? I said to him, "My God, John, they're going to be a hard audience. They're too busy talking to hear a word Peter is saying."

'John just said, "They'll listen to *me*."

'I was astonished at how calm he was. I shouldn't have been. John stood up and from his first words he held those people in the palm of his hand. They heard him out in total silence, except when they were laughing their heads off as he told his inspirational stories and jokes, and at the end they gave him a great ovation.

'John sat down, grinned, and said, "Told ya they'd listen to me!" He was confident, composed, articulate and really funny. I'd never realised he had this gift.'

Motivational Speaking

I do two kinds of public speaking: motivational talks and stand-up comedy. Occasionally I combine the two.

With the former, I talk about the lessons I've learned playing and coaching rugby league. I also draw on the wisdom of the great coaches I've played under and those, like Vince Lombardi, whose methods I've read deeply about.

Basically, my message is that you can learn a lot about life from playing sport. I believe that sport is a valuable and challenging activity in which a young participant learns self-control, and gains self-respect and self-esteem. To succeed at sport a player must make a tremendous effort, make sacrifices, while abiding by the rules, considering the rights of others and staying within the bounds of decency and sportsmanship.

Coaching, I say, is an honourable and dignified profession in which you can have a major effect on your players' mental and physical development and attitudes and give them standards that they can live by for the rest of their lives. If a coach can help a young player to have a purpose in life, to set worthwhile goals, if a coach can help a young person to fully realise their potential, then that coach will have made a wonderful contribution to society.

Sports, such as rugby league, are only games – but they are important. If you take all the ingredients of a football match, put them in a barrel, stir them up and tip them out, you'll have a well-proportioned phase of the Australian way of life.

My Life in Stand-up

My fully-fledged career as a comedian grew out of a few invitations Arthur and I received to be guests at sporting functions around Sydney and in the bush after our ABC stint. We'd get a good roll-up because people always like a laugh, especially if it's that great, dry Australian humour, laconic and understated and a bit outrageous. And they love Arthur, who of course is a legend. They really appreciate him in Queensland, in his home town of Roma, and in places like Emerald, Moranbah and Bluff in central Queensland, where the miners come determined to have the time of their life. There are few better feelings than to walk into a hall and find it packed with people eagerly anticipating your show. And when they laugh and clap it's really great.

After I gave a show at the Iron Horse Inn at Cardiff in May 1993, a local league-lover and amateur poet, Lindsay Young, presented me with a laminated poster as a thank-you. On it was an ode to me, titled 'The Bomber'.

Early on, when we appeared as a double act, Arthur and I would tell a few footy stories about our playing days, usually ad-libbed and all a bit rough and ready. Then gradually over time, as I became more confident standing up and speaking in front of a crowd, I spent a bit of time planning what I'd say and the jokes I'd tell. Fashioning my material to suit my audience. I memorised hundreds of jokes and yarns, so I could drop them into my act when appropriate. To hone my timing and delivery – so important to a stand-up comedian – I listened time and again to the cassette tapes of experienced comedians.

Material was never a problem. I became good at creating jokes based on footy, human foibles and current events. I was not above pinching a joke and adapting it. And it's a curse and a blessing for everyone who tells jokes to be swamped after the show by punters saying, 'Hey, have you heard the one about …?' Usually these offerings are pretty average, but occasionally a bloke will drop a gem on you, and your repertoire is instantly enriched.

'The Bomber' by Lindsay Young

Mid-January 1946, Queensland, Atherton
This town was the birthplace of a Peard son christened John.
The family moved to New South Wales and young John played
    the game
Of rugby league ... and played it well and made himself a name

At 19 Peardy made the grade in '66 at Easts
Six years till '71 a Rooster ... experience increased
'72 he switched to St George for the next two seasons
Then back to Easts for two more years and not without good reason

For Easts compiled a super side and won the title twice
With John Peard as a vital link, and then he was enticed
To Parramatta and his tactical kick, the bomb
A pinpoint-accurate up-and-under, Peard made it belong

Four years with Parramatta, '76 to '79
He bombed teams to oblivion, he drove 'em off their mind
A stylish five-eighth with good hands, rock solid in defence
A pivot in the classic mould with great resilience

A groin injury which would not heal would force him from the
    game
Eight times he'd worn Australia's green and gold, achieving fame
He joined the coaching ranks with Parramatta 1980
'82 and '83 at Penrith ... mostly the rep scene lately

In '86 and '90 City teams were his domain
And '88 with New South Wales, he held the Origin reins
1990 assistant coach to Gibson with the Blues
Since then, assistant coach at Easts ... John Peard has paid
    his dues

Some former sportsmen don't bother to prepare their performances when they address an audience. They think it's enough to bask in their former glory, just cop the money and get up on stage, take questions from the audience and ad-lib the answers.

Putting a lot of effort and time into my preparation before a speaking engagement was the least I could do. The audiences were salt-of-the-earth people, sport lovers, sometimes blokes I'd played with and against, and they were genuinely interested in hearing me and afterwards getting to shake my hand in the bar. I'd arrive at the venue an hour before I was to speak and ask the organisers things like 'Who's that bloke with the red nose over there?', 'Can you point out to me the neighbourhood SP bookie?', 'What's the local copper's name?' and 'How did the local team go on the weekend?' – so I could drop little yarns about colourful locals, or if the footy team had been flogged on the weekend I'd rub that in a bit. Occasionally I'd inject some current affairs into my yarns to keep things topical.

If I was talking at, say, St George Leagues Club, I'd do my homework on the great Saints heroes such as Norm Provan, Chook Raper, Poppa Clay and Reg Gasnier. On the night it might go like this:

> 'Reg Gasnier, what a champion. But did you know there was only one bloke he feared. The huge and hard-tackling Great Britain winger Billy Boston. It's true. Billy used to wait till Harry Wells passed Reg the ball and then tear in from his wing like a runaway truck and smash poor Reg. Reg got cleaned up like this on numerous occasions until he finally worked out a way to stop Billy. I asked Reg about it one day and he was

happy to explain: "Well, Bomber, first I'd concentrate on catching the ball when Harry passed it to me. Then, just when I saw Billy looming, I'd bend down and pick up a handful of shit and then I'd throw that shit right in Billy's face."

"But Reg, what if there's shit on the field?"

"Bomber," said Reg, "when Billy Boston comes at you, *there'll* be shit."'

Sometimes Artie and I were a double act, kind of like an ocker version of Laurel and Hardy or Abbott and Costello. He was the straight man, laying the platform for my punchlines. Occasionally my co-comedian was Noel Kelly, the fiery Wests prop of the '50s and '60s whom I'd admired so much when I was starting out.

'Ned,' I'd say, 'you were always getting sent off, weren't you?'

'I was, Bomber,' Ned would riposte, right on cue (after we'd rehearsed it about a hundred times). 'Even today, long after I've retired, when the mailman blows his whistle I head straight for the shower!'

Other times I appeared solo, as myself or doing my Hoges impersonation, with the usual get-up: footy jumper and stubbies, Newtown footy socks, boots and an outrageously bad blond wig.

On the Road

I began getting up on stage in the early '90s and still do it today, in spite of being a bit hampered by my stroke. I don't charge a fee to appear, just my transport costs to get to the venue, and if it's in the bush, the cost of a room at a country pub. In my fifteen years or more of speaking engagements I must have played most of the clubs in New South Wales and Queensland.

Arthur and I also visited Papua New Guinea, where they truly love their rugby league, and to Manila in the Philippines, where Graeme Langlands had a nightclub for a while.

Arthur and I and the Melbourne Cup–winning jockey Larry Olsen were invited to speak at a sportsmen's lunch at one Manila club, and Changa and scores of other expats rolled up to hear us. Now, there's nothing sleazier than a nightclub in daytime. You can see the grubbiness, vermin and the rubbish lying everywhere that the darkness of the evening conceals. It's terrible. The club had strippers performing, and they lose their allure, too, in the harsh light of day. The girls were dancing, miming, singing karaoke and, unfortunately, that's not all they did. Arthur, Larry and I had to get up and speak after a stripper who smoked a cigarette with her private parts. Talk about a hard act to follow!

Arthur said, 'Bomber, what are we going to do? We're history. No one's going to want to listen to us after that!'

'Go over and grab Larry by the collar and the crotch of his pants and throw him up onto the stage,' I suggested. 'He can break the ice, and then when the crowd have forgotten the stripper we'll get up and knock 'em dead.'

Arthur did as I said, picked up little Larry and slung him onto the stage. Poor Larry. He's a good bloke and can be a funny man, but his jokes fell flat. When we had our turn, we were too.

We had better luck in Australia. I've always looked forward to my outback tours. You meet people you'd never expect to bump into. At Moranbah, a tiny Queensland town of demountable buildings that exists for the local mine, I was sitting in the makeshift TAB watching the screens when someone belted me on the back. I swung around. It was Chook Raper.

'Chook!' I said in surprise, 'What are you doing here?'

'Selling mine chemicals for Bozo Fulton,' he explained.

'Arthur and I are doing a show here tonight at the club. Why not come?'

Chook, who'd attend the opening of an envelope, and has been known to page himself at a club so everyone knows he's there and can see him striding across the auditorium to take care of his important business, was at the club three hours before Artie and me.

Roasting Arthur

They say if you steal jokes from one comedian it's stealing, but if you pilfer from ten it's research. I first heard the next two jokes from the great Brian Doyle and use them shamelessly, slightly modified, particularly when travelling around with Arthur Beetson. Arthur was the perfect fall guy in my jokes.

> You know, folks, you get a chance to really know a bloke when you're sitting alongside him in a car for six or seven hours. On our way here today, I got a bit philosophical with the big bloke.
>
> 'Arthur,' I said, 'what would you do if you knew you had only had thirty minutes to live?'
>
> He said, 'I'd make love to the first thing that moved. What would you do, Bomber?'
>
> I said, 'Arthur, I wouldn't move for thirty minutes.'

> 'Friends, did you realise that big Artie here is a very religious fella? In fact, he talks to the Almighty every day. Last week Arthur asked God, 'How long is a million years to you, O Lord?'

God replied, 'A million years to me is just like a single second is to you.'

Then Artie asked, 'Lord, what is a million dollars to you?'

The Almighty said, 'A million dollars to me is just like a penny is to you.'

So Arthur summoned up all his courage. 'O Lord, can I have one of your pennies?'

Said God, 'Certainly, Arthur, just a second.'

Ladies and gentlemen, Arthur is a very generous bloke. You may not know this, but he and I have a foster child in the Philippines, a dear little boy from a poor background, and last year we sent the kid a photo of ourselves. Now he sends *us* twenty dollars a month!'

I loved to give Arthur a roasting, especially over his weight.

Arthur used to be an all-round athlete, now he's just all round.

He lost fifteen kilos, but he'll find 'em.

When Arthur visits my place it doesn't matter what room he's in, he's always right next to me.

If Artie wants a hangover he only needs to sit on a stool.

Arthur was going to have a facelift, but the crane broke.

I drove Artie to Newcastle in my Toyota and when he got out, the *car* jumped in the air.

Arthur went to confession and said to the priest, 'I've spent all morning looking at my naked body in the mirror and thinking how good I look. Will I have to do penance, Father?'

'No, Arthur,' said the priest, 'you only do penance for a sin, not a mistake.'

Artie hung his undies on the line and squatters moved in.

Arthur is an incredibly intelligent guy, but that never stopped me from sledging him.

Arthur met a girl in a nightclub. He took her home in his car and put the hard word on her. She said, 'I'd love to Artie, but I've got my menstrual cycle.' He replied, 'No problem, love. Put it in the boot.'

Arthur burned his feet cooking spaghetti. It was in a can and the label read: 'Place in saucepan and stand in boiling water for eight minutes.'

When he was growing up in Roma, Arthur had to help prepare the Christmas feast. 'Mum,' he'd say, 'I've plucked and stuffed the turkey. All you have to do is kill it and cook it!'

Politically Incorrect

Sometimes a joke is close to the bone, but no less funny for that, and at the right place at the right time with the right audience you can just about get away with irreverent humour. I have no trouble telling slightly blue jokes, nothing as X-rated as some other comedians tell, but ones that may be considered a little risqué.

Yet I never lapsed into bad taste when I knew Jack Gibson was out there in the crowd. As Mark Harris learned back in the Red Faces days, Jack hates dirty yarns. Once I came down off the stage and he said, shaking his head, 'Peard, you said "shit" twice tonight.' Another time at Parramatta I was giving a talk and a few questionable words crept in and Jack barked from second row, 'Bomber, there's never been a speech too short.' This was a verbal kick in the pants for me, his way of telling me to clean up my act. His words echoed his old coaching edict: 'Bomber, there's never been a kick too high.'

The Key to Heaven

Religious jokes have the potential to upset people, but I've never really had a problem with this one, which I found on the internet:

Former US president Bill Clinton and the Pope die on the same day, and due to an administrative stuff-up, serial philanderer Clinton lands in Heaven and the clean-living, God-fearing Pope in Hell. The Pope explains the situation to the Hell administration, they check their paperwork and the error is acknowledged. They explain, however, that it will take twenty-four hours to make the switch.

The next day, the Pope is called in and the Hell administration bids him farewell and he heads for Heaven. On the way up, he meets Clinton coming down.

The Pope says, 'Hello Bill, sorry about the mix-up.'

'No problem,' says Clinton.

'Well,' continues the Pope, 'I'm really excited about going to Heaven.'

Clinton says, 'Why's that?'

'All my life I've wanted to meet the Virgin Mary,' says the Pope.

Says Clinton, 'You're a day late!'

My Mate, Matthew Mitric

Any comedian or speaker will tell you he lives for applause and to see people out there in the audience laughing their head off. Sometimes the rewards are even greater.

I met Matthew Mitric at Balmain Leagues Club in the late 1990s when I was master of ceremonies at a fundraising auction for children's cancer. Matthew was a little boy who had a rare type of blood cancer. He and his mother had come to hear me speak and be part of the occasion. During the afternoon I saw him sitting in the audience and went down to say hi to him and his mother, Kim. We became friends and I took Matt under my wing. He was a mighty little bloke who loved footy, and especially the Bulldogs.

I said to him, 'Have a look at all the gear up there on the stage and whatever you want, I'll buy it for you.' He chose a football signed by every Canterbury-Bankstown star. Steve Edge was auctioneer and I said, 'Edgey, this little bloke down the front has cancer and he wants the Bulldogs ball. When I put my hand up for it, knock it down to me. I don't care who else is bidding. That's ball's mine.'

Signed balls normally go for around sixty dollars, but when Steve reached twenty he said, 'Peardy's bidding. Twenty dollars! Going once, twice, three times ... to Bomber Peard!'

Kim was sole carer for Matthew, and his sister Danielle, at their home at Umina on the New South Wales central coast. The family was doing it tough, emotionally and financially, so I would ring and write to them often, and drive up to drop in for a chat and to give Matthew football gear and pressies.

Around 2000, when Matthew was clearly going downhill, Kim called me and said he really wanted to have a ride in my concrete truck. So next Sunday I went to the plant, picked up the truck and drove it up the freeway to Umina. We beetled all over town and he laughed and clapped when I let him spray the truck's water hose.

I bought Matthew a trail bike and thought I'd surprise him by leaving it under his house. When I was stashing it where he'd easily find it I saw he already had a trail bike, a much better model than the one I'd purchased. I left the new bike there anyway, and called Kim and told her to sell it and keep whatever money she could get for it to help pay the heavy medical bills.

I'm no saint, far from it, but that suffering family meant a lot to me. I like to think that my times with the Mitrics proved that I'd come a long way from the self-absorbed and selfish bloke I'd been in younger days.

An Audience with John Peard

For anyone who hasn't seen me in action at one of my speaking engagements, I've been taping my performances so I can present for you here a pretty typical show. Feel free to use any of the jokes whenever you like.

> I'm John Peard, I'm an alcoholic, I think I'm at the wrong meeting! Well, anyway folks, thanks for inviting me here tonight. A great American gridiron coach once said that every time you lose you die a little. Well, I coached New South Wales to a three–nil series loss, and I coached Penrith when wins were few and far between. So believe me, folks, I'm *really* glad to be here.

I have a thousand wife jokes, which always go down well ...

Ladies and gentlemen, I wish you knew my wife. Ours is a marriage made in heaven. We got hitched because God didn't mean humans to be happy all their life.

Last week we had our anniversary. I said, 'Darling, what would you like for your anniversary?'

'A divorce,' she said.

'Oh, I wasn't thinking of spending that much.'

I was driving with my wife in Queensland when a cop pulled us over. The missus is hard of hearing. The cop said, 'I'm giving you a ticket for speeding, mate.'

My wife said, 'What'd he saaay?' I told her, 'Darling, he said he's going to give me a speeding ticket.'

Then the policeman said, 'Driver, I've clocked you at 120 kilometres an hour, and you're lucky I don't run you in.'

Said my wife, 'What'd he saaay?' 'Darling, he said I was doing 120 kilometres an hour and I'm lucky he isn't going to arrest me.'

The cop went on, 'Sir, can I see your driver's licence?' I gave it to him. He looked at it and remarked, 'Oh, you're from Cairns ... I went to Cairns once, and I had the worst sex I've ever had in my life.'

My wife said, 'What'd he saaay?' I said, 'Darling, he says he knows you.'

I asked my wife what she wanted for her birthday and she replied, 'A widow's pension.'

My wife said to me, 'Darling, take me somewhere I've never been.' I took her to the kitchen.

My wife gave birth, and the baby was, well, dark-skinned. The doctor said to me, 'Sir, are sure this baby is yours?'

I said, 'Probably ... she burns everything else!'

My wife asked me if I knew what an erogenous zone was. I said, 'Sure, I got booked in one this morning!'

I saw my ex-wife at a party last night and we got on so well I said, 'Darlin', why don't we go back to my place and make love?' She replied, 'Over my dead body!'

'So,' I said, 'you haven't changed.'

My wife took a photo of my penis the other day. I asked her, 'Dearest, are you going to stick the picture in our family album?'

She said, 'No, I'm going to get it enlarged.'

I'm not proud to say that things got so bad in the sack with my wife that to get a thrill I was reduced to making calls to one of those phone numbers where a woman talks dirty to you. Funny isn't it, folks, that if a man talks dirty to a woman it's sexual harassment, if a woman does the same to a man it's $9.95 a minute?

My wife and I have a fairly normal marriage. The other day she and I went to Taronga Park Zoo and when we were strolling past the gorilla cage, this huge ape stuck his paw through the bars and pulled her into his cage. He was about to have his way with her.

My wife screamed, 'John, do something!'

I said, 'Tell him about your migraine!'

I got home late the other night after a big night on the booze with the blokes. My missus said, 'What are you doing getting home at this time?'

I told her, 'This is the only place that's still open.'

She noticed that my wallet was empty and said, 'Where's all your money? What have you done with it?'

'Darling, I bought something for the house.'

'What?'

'A round of drinks.'

I phoned the doctor. 'Doc, I'm worried about my wife. She thinks she's a horse. Could you have a look at her?'

The doctor said, 'Mr Peard, this could be a long and costly treatment.'

'Money's no object, doc,' I said. 'She's won her first three races."

I staggered home last night at 3 am, as full as a goog. I woke my wife. 'Darling, it's miraculous! It's unbelievable! I just went for a leak and when I started a light came on, and when I finished it went off! It's a miracle!'

'No it's not,' said my wife. 'You just pissed in the refrigerator.'

My wife's so plain, she couldn't lure a bloke out of a burning building!

My wife went to the zoo and had to buy two tickets. One to get in and one to get out!

My wife talks through her nose. She's worn her mouth out.

Fore! Golf is a gift for comedians ...

I used to play every Saturday at Woolooware in a foursome with Jack Gibson, Ron Massey and an old bloke named Bill. Sadly, Bill passed away not long ago. Nothing serious wrong with him, he just died. We missed Bill, because out of all of us he was the only one still with 20/20 vision and he could tell Jack, Ron and me where our balls had landed.

At Bill's funeral, Jack said to Barry Bent, the pro at the golf club, 'Barry, you've got to get us another golf partner to replace Bill by next weekend. We need someone to tell us where our balls go, someone with 20/20 vision.' Barry said not to worry, he had someone in mind.

The following Saturday we rolled up at Woolooware and Jack said to Barry, 'So, did you get us a partner?'

'Sure did, Jack, I got you old Charlie over there.'

Jack looked over and said, 'You're kidding, Barry. Charlie's ninety-seven!'

Barry replied, 'He might be ninety-seven, Jack, but he's got 20/20 vision. He'll tell you where your balls go.' Jack looked doubtful, but said, 'Come on then Charlie, up to the tee.'

We all hit off. Jack squared away and whacked a screamer. 'Charlie,' he said, 'did you see where that went?'

Charlie said, 'Yeah.'

Jack said, 'Well, where is it?'

Charlie said, 'I forget.'

Did you hear about the two golfers who played a lot together? One had a terrible hook and he was always hitting his ball into a water hazard or clear out of the course and onto the road. His mate finally said to him, 'You've got a nasty hook there.'

The other bloke said, 'So you've noticed, have you?'

'Yes, I used to have a hook like that, but I cured it.'

'How?'

'I made love to my wife every morning for three weeks. Cured my hook just like that! You should consider it.' The other bloke looked thoughtful.

Anyway, three-and-a-half weeks later, they played together again. The fellow with the hook got up to the tee and hit his ball beautifully, straight as a gun barrel down the fairway and right onto the putting green. His partner leaned on his club and said, 'So, I see you've fixed your hook. Did you take my advice?'

'As a matter of fact I did,' said his friend. 'And by the way, you've got a lovely bedroom.'

And what about the man and wife who played together all the time, and one day as they walked between the tee and the hole she said to him, 'Darling, if I died, would you get married again?'

'Well, love, if you passed away and if I ever met someone and fell in love with her like I fell in love with you, I suppose I would remarry.'

'Would you let your new wife live in our house?'

'Well, love, I'm in no financial position to buy any more real estate, particularly around this way, so I guess she'd have to live in our house.'

'You would, eh?' said the wife. 'And, tell me, would you play golf with her?'

'You know I love my golf, darling, so I probably would play with her.'

'Would you let her use my clubs?' 'Shit no,' said the husband, 'she's left-handed.'

Old footy-playing friends and foes are fair game ...

One old team-mate is the stingiest bloke I've ever known. Though, in fairness, once he did buy five of us a beer; problem was, we wanted one each ...

Another time a good mate of ours died. We went to the funeral home and there was old Billy lying in his open coffin. John Quayle and I thought we'd abide by the old tradition and send Billy to heaven with a bit of ready cash in case he needed it on his celestial journey. We each pinned a $100 note on his chest.

Our stingy friend saw what we'd done and, not wanting to be left out, responded in magnificent fashion. He reached into his pocket for his chequebook, wrote a cheque for $300, plonked it on Billy's shirtfront and stuck John's and my cash in his pocket.

Sometimes I take hoary testicle jokes and give them a footy spin ...

Back when I was playing with the Roosters there was no such thing as a full-time professional footballer. We all had to have jobs. We needed the money and, besides, Jack Gibson insisted on it. So one day a bunch of us went up to Waverley Council to find work. I said to the employment officer, 'We're Easts first graders and we've come for a job, mate.'

The officer said, 'I don't care who you blokes are. To get a job with Waverley Council you have to pass a medical test conducted by our doctor.'

'Oh come on, mate,' I said, 'we're first-grade footballers and fit as bulls.'

'You may be, but our by-laws make it very clear that to be eligible for a job you have to pass the medical. Take the test or scram.'

He had us over a barrel, so we got our gear off and prepared to front the doc. I went into the clinic first and the doctor felt my balls and said, 'You're OK, Peard, you can work for the council. Clock on at 7 am Monday.'

My team-mates all passed, too, and received the same message. 'Start work at 7 on Monday morning.'

Finally, the last bloke went in – he'll remain nameless for reasons that will become obvious – and the doctor had a feel of his privates. 'What the …?' the doc said in astonishment. 'You've got no testicles!'

'No,' said the player, 'I've never had any. Does that mean I can't work for Waverley Council?'

'Of course you can,' replied the medic, 'only you'll start on Monday at 9 am.'

'But the other blokes start at 7!'

Said the doc, 'They do mate, but you've seen council workers. For the first two hours on the job all they do is stand around scratching their balls!'

Well, my job at the council didn't last long. I tried to get a position in an orange juice factory, but I couldn't concentrate so they canned me. Then I worked in the woods as a lumberjack but I couldn't cut it and they gave me the axe. After that I tried to be a tailor, but I just wasn't suited for it. Next, I got a job in an auto muffler factory, but that was exhausting. So I joined a swimming pool maintenance firm only to find the work was too draining. Next I became a professional fisherman, until I discovered I couldn't live on my net income. A health club hired me but let me go. They reckoned I wasn't fit for the job. I finally became a historian until I realised there was no future in it.

And folks, as you know, State of Origin, with all the close scores we've had over the years, is a game of inches. And that reminds me of the time when US President Richard Nixon was welcoming all the troops back from Vietnam in 1968. He met the soldiers as they disembarked from the plane, and beside him was a helper with medals in a beautiful carved wooden box. As each man came down the steps, Tricky Dicky would pin a medal on the bloke's chest. Suddenly the helper looked panic-stricken. 'Mr President, we've run out of medals!'

Always at his best in a crisis, Nixon said, 'Don't worry, son. We'll give the rest of the guys some money instead. That'll keep 'em happy.' So he got the fellas without medals together and explained, 'Guys, I want to thank you for what you did over there in Vietnam. We've no medals left, but to show my, and your country's, appreciation, what I'd like to do is measure a part of your anatomy – any part you care to nominate – and however long it is, we'll pay the same number of thousands of dollars.'

The first serviceman in the line was a little fat bloke. Nixon asked him, 'And, soldier, which of your body parts would you like us to measure?'

He replied, 'My stomach, President Nixon.'

They put a tape around the guy: 48 inches. Said Nixon, 'Give that man $48,000!'

Next in line was a tall, skinny bloke. Said the President, 'What do you want us to measure, sonny?'

'My height, Mr Nixon.'

He was 84 inches tall. 'Give that man $84,000,' said the President.

Then came a little fellow, 65 centimetres tall and weighing 22 kilos. Nixon whispered to his offsider, 'This guy won't cost us much!' Then he turned to the tiny chap and said, 'Now, what do you want us to measure?'

'Sir, I want you to measure from the end of my penis back to my testicles.'

'Oh come on, son, that's no good, you'll only get a few bucks. After all you've done for the United States you're entitled to a reasonable payout.'

The soldier was adamant. 'That's what I want, Mr President.'

'Well, OK,' said President Nixon, 'measure him up.' The helper pulled down the soldier's pants and Nixon gasped in shock. 'But you've got no testicles! Where are they?'

'Sir, they're back in Vietnam!'

CHAPTER 14

Stroke Victim

I Should Have Died

In 2002, I was fifty-seven but felt forty years younger. Not for a moment did I consider myself a potential stroke victim. I was having too much fun, and I knew I was going to live forever. I slogged away by day driving my concrete truck and rewarded myself by night and on weekends by leading the life of Riley.

After I parked the truck each afternoon I'd typically head off to North Cronulla surf club's gym to pump iron, have a run and a swim, then have four or five schooners of beer with my mate Peter Cruikshank and a few other blokes before going home around 8 pm to cook a hearty meal and flop into bed by 10. I'd do a speaking gig once a week or fortnight. Weekends comprised more weight-lifting, more running and swimming, drinking, the races on Saturday, and going to see the Roosters or the Sharks on Sunday. I couldn't see things changing drastically, and that suited me. One thing I realise, in hindsight: I was complacent, living in a lotus land of my own making, and I had pretty much abandoned my lifelong habit of setting goals for myself. I was happy to drift.

When I was invited by BHP Blue Scope to go to Brisbane for three days during State of Origin week, to share the stage at footy club and casino functions with Graeme Langlands, John Raper and Reg Gasnier, I leapt at the opportunity. As I knew we would, we knocked ourselves around up there. Each day was a beer-fuelled party that started early and finished late. Much of that time away is a blur. Jeez, we put some ale away, and we kept drinking on the plane almost right to the moment we landed at Sydney airport in the late morning of 6 June.

Well, you know what happened on 7 June. I could have died. I should have died. Doctors agreed that a less fit man would have passed away in the night. There was no guarantee, my loved ones were told, that I'd survive the day, or the week.

The head of emergency at the hospital told a devastated Peter Cruikshank, who ran the coffee shop at the hospital, that there was a strong chance I would not survive: 'I know he's a determined bloke, but this is a real bad one.' When Peter expressed amazement that someone as fit as me could suffer a stroke, the doctor told him that heavy exercise performed by someone with hypertension or heart disease can cause strains that lead to strokes; and often it wasn't the likely suspects, the couch potatoes and the junk-food eaters, who suffered strokes because they never exerted themselves. It was the people who thought they were indestructible and never had check-ups. That was me to a T.

As the medical staff worked desperately to save my life, I lay there in a daze. I was in no pain, but dizzy and completely uncoordinated. The doctors told me I was lucky to be alive because I had suffered a major stroke after a dissection in my carotid artery affected the right-hand side of my brain and so incapacitated my left side from head to toe. The hard partying and the weight-lifting hadn't helped. Then they gave me the third degree. They asked if there was a history of stroke in my family, if I had cholesterol or high blood pressure, diabetes or any kind of heart disease. They needed to know if I was a heavy drinker, if I smoked. The deadly seriousness of my predicament sank in. I was in terrible trouble.

To try to figure out the cause of my stroke the team in intensive care gave me a CT scan, which showed them a picture of the condition of the right and left hemispheres of my brain, the brain stem and the cerebellum. I was taken in an ambulance to Sutherland Hospital where the doctors performed an angiogram to check the state of my blood vessels. X-ray dye was injected through a catheter in my groin into my bloodstream. As it coursed through my body, they could follow its progress on a screen, and see whether there were blockages in the vessels of my brain, lungs, abdomen, arms and legs.

Then, to prevent a follow-up stroke, they gave me medication to relax me and thin my blood and to dissolve any blood clots in my system that could worm their way to my damaged brain. They lowered my cholesterol and blood pressure.

'Bomber, a Stroke? Never!'

As I lay at death's door, word spread that I'd had a stroke. Loved ones and friends told me later that they were incredulous. 'Bomber, a stroke? Never!'

They came in droves, but in those dangerous early days, only family and my closest friends were allowed in to see me. My daughters Johanna and Amanda came, and Christine. My sisters Margaret and Di and their husbands, Peter Moscatt and Robert Conneeley, and brother Geoffrey. My father, Jack, though in his early nineties by this time, came too. My great friend and girlfriend Jo Richards showed up. Peter Cruikshank and Keiran Speed sat with me. So did Artie Beetson, Bob McMillan, Graham Bowen and Fred Pagano and more. They say I wasn't a pretty sight.

Margaret remembers coming into the ward to see me that first day, about ten hours after I'd been admitted. Chris, Amanda and Johanna, who was heavily pregnant, were already there and they took Margaret aside and gave her the news straight, that the doctors had told them that they didn't know if I was going to last the night. Margaret burst into tears, and they kept repeating, 'He's *not* going to die. He's *not* going to die ... It's just that we don't know what his chances of rehabilitation are.'

I can't remember a thing about how I was that night, but Margaret assures me I was lying there quietly on my right side, holding on to the edge of the bed. She kissed me and asked how I was, and apparently I replied, 'Oh, I've got a bit of a headache, but otherwise fine thanks mate.'

Riding a Rollercoaster

Margaret returned to my bedside a couple of weeks later, when it seemed pretty certain that I'd pull through but they still didn't know the extent of the stroke's effect on me. She says I was remote towards her, listening to music through headphones, that I seemed depressed and uncommunicative. I hardly acknowledged her and took off my headphones only long enough to say a curt hello. Again, I have only blurry memories, but I have no doubt Margaret is telling the truth. I was riding a rollercoaster that lurched between hope, frustration and depression.

Everybody, my family and the friends who came to visit me, bore the brunt of my tangled emotions. In my stricken state I wondered what the hell had happened to me, Mr Bulletproof. Strokes and heart attacks happened to other people. Not Bomber Peard. I was bewildered and distraught. I felt helpless. My life was in the hands of others. My emotions ran the gamut. At times I laughed with my visitors or at a TV show or a joke someone sent me. I was occasionally irrational and moody. Other times I despaired, and sometimes I wept.

Hopefully, I was mostly nice to be around. After I was moved off the critical list and out of intensive care into a regular ward, the seat next to my bed never had a chance to get cold. My Brisbane partners in crime, Graeme Langlands, John Raper and Reg Gasnier, visited. So did Steve Mortimer and Harry Eden. My old coach from Bondi United, Curly Simons. Old Roosters such as Les Hayes, Bunny Reilly, Graham Mayhew and John Mayes rolled up, and Saints and Eels team-mates. Some of the blokes I'd coached at Penrith fronted, such as big Darryl Brohman, who always seemed to arrive when the hospital tucker was being served. One day I opened my eyes and Tony Quirk, the St George fullback whom I'd tormented with my bombs all those years ago, was there at my bedside. Today, as I remember Tony's kindness, tears come to my eyes. Jack Gibson turned up twice a week. 'What's doin', kid?' he'd say in his laconic way. 'Anything new?'

So many people came to see me that the hospital staff had to restrict the numbers. They were turning people away and asking if it would be OK if they came back later.

Bobby McMillan, a former Rabbitoh and my weight-lifting partner, would encourage me: 'Come on, Bomber. Try to move your toe. Just a tiny bit. You can do it!' Bobby, in his way, was giving me rehab.

I also owe a debt to many people I didn't know, such as radio's Ray Hadley and members of the public who remembered my playing days, who sent me messages of hope and inspiration. One person sent me a poem, the first stanza went:

See Bomber flashing through the town
Lithe and light and golden brown
Broad of shoulders, slim of hips
Words of wisdom on his lips
It's an honour to get a nod
From Bomber the Mighty! Bomber the God!

I appreciated the poem, but right then I felt anything but mighty or like a God!

In my less lucid moments I introduced my visitors to 'Reg Gasnier', the bloke in the next bed. Heavens knows what the real Reg thought when he dropped in to see me and I introduced him to himself. I asked a nurse why I was convinced the poor bloke beside me was Gasnier, and she said, 'John, you're hallucinating. Something major has happened to your brain and it's doing things it normally doesn't. It'll pass.'

The love of my family and the deep concern of my mates spurred me to get better. Scarcely one visitor left my bedside without saying, 'Bomber, if anyone can get over something like this, mate, you can.' Each day the hospital orderly brought in scores of get-well cards.

Like most of us, I had little idea what a stroke was. A heart attack perhaps? Something that derailed the central nervous system. In the months and years that followed my 'brain attack', for that's what the medicos call a stroke, I learned plenty about this terrible condition that lays low around 53,000 Australians every year.

Australia's National Stroke Foundation is a marvellous organisation that has helped many thousands of stroke survivors and those who share their lives. They explained to me that stroke is the second largest cause of death and a leading cause of disability among Australian adults. Of the 53,000 who suffer a stroke each year, one-third will not survive the first twelve months. At the end of the book the Australian Stroke Foundation explains the condition in detail, and their advice is well worth reading, but briefly, stroke is a cardiovascular disease that affects the arteries leading to the brain and within it. A stroke is suffered when a blood vessel that is transporting nutrients and oxygen to the brain is blocked by a clot, or bursts. A brain deprived of blood and oxygen begins to die.

My stroke, I believe, came out of the blue, but the Stroke Foundation advises that generally there are warning signs that you are about to suffer a stroke. These include weakness or numbness of the face, leg, arm or sides; difficulty in speaking or understanding what others are saying; dizziness, loss of vision or blurred vision; severe headache; difficulty swallowing.

Age, gender and a family history of strokes can make you a candidate. And my combination of drinking and lifting heavy weights definitely made me susceptible. Also, according to the Stroke Foundation, if you have any of the following conditions, you could be too: high blood pressure; a smoking habit, high cholesterol; poor diet; an aversion to exercise; obesity, diabetes; drink too much alcohol; have heart problems. The good news is that many of the preceding risk factors can be controlled or eliminated. If you're worried, see a doctor. If this book achieves nothing else than sending a reader to a medico who saves his or her life it will have been worthwhile.

A Fight for Rehab

Unbeknown to me a battle was raging over my recovery. The prognosis was not good and medical opinion on my future was divided. Even if I survived now, there was a view a second, probably fatal, stroke was pretty certain sooner rather than later, and even if I avoided that and lived, I'd be a virtual vegetable. Margaret, her husband Peter, Chris, Amanda and Johanna and my brother Geoff had a meeting at the hospital to discuss my prognosis.

There was a body of opinion that opposed rehab therapy. 'John has had a very serious stroke,' said one expert present. 'He had a blockage in his carotid artery and the loss of blood to his brain has destroyed part of his brain. Those damaged parts may never recover. He has lost half of his sight in each eye. He may never be able to comprehend even the simplest processes. He may never even be able to make himself a cup of tea or find his way from point A to point B.'

A nursing home was suggested and rehab appeared out of the question.

Of course, the doom-laden prognosis brought out the old headmistress in my sister, and she towelled up the doctor.

Margaret remembers a heated encounter.

'How can you say that about my brother?' she exploded. 'Surely it's your responsibility to offer rehabilitation. You don't know John. He's been a champion footballer, and has fought all his life. You don't know his fighting qualities. Think of the very best outcome you can for John, and I guarantee that he will exceed it. I'm sure you absolutely have very good medical knowledge but you're not dealing with just anyone here. You're dealing with somebody who has always, always, always succeeded.'

'Well,' Margaret continued, 'he *is* having rehab, and if you won't give it to him, I'll find someone who will. Please, won't you just follow his progress for the next four weeks and make your decision then?'

It was finally agreed that this would happen.

Then, Margaret, Peter, my daughters, and Christine, who in spite of our no longer being together dropped everything to come to my aid, read everything about strokes they could lay their hands on, and they began calling around to see what rehab options were available. Margaret rang every doctor she knew and all the doctors her friends knew. They all spent huge amounts of time on the phone, to hospitals, clinics and rehab centres all around Sydney. It would be expensive, even with my private health insurance, but it brings me to tears even today to tell you that there wasn't one of them who wouldn't have hocked their home to help me pay for the treatment.

Margaret says that while it was a terrible time when Mum died, those four weeks when my future hung in the balance was the worst experience of her life. She'd wake each morning and think, 'This can't be happening. Not to John, the man who could do anything. Who had been indestructible since we were kids together.' She had no doubt that if I had the chance to get better, through rehab, I'd make it.

At 6 pm on the last day of the allotted four weeks, the hospital called Margaret and said, 'Mrs Moscatt, we've decided John can have rehabilitation treatment. Starting right away.'

The day I entered the rehabilitation ward at Sutherland Hospital was a red letter day for me. I was so proud as I wheeled my wheelchair into the ward. With my disability it was a huge effort, and it exhausted me just to make that chair go straight. My family and my physiotherapist were all there to see me, and I could see the pride in their eyes, too.

'This Bloody Stroke Won't Beat Me'

Rehab was the blessing we knew it would be. The staff were magnificent. Nothing was too much trouble for them. They made me do those exercises every day, guiding me, inspiring me, haranguing me, and day by day, week by week, month by month, I improved. By two months into the treatment, a little movement and feeling had returned to my left side.

For the next four months I did rehab at Sutherland Hospital. Each day at 10.30 am I'd drag myself out of bed and into my wheelchair, and wheel myself from my ward to the rehab section. After a while I was able to avoid slamming into the walls. I got to know all the nurses in rehab, and flirted with them outrageously. My sense of humour began to return.

There were many exercises and routines they put me through. One was to lie on my back and lift my left leg slowly up and down, then roll over onto my stomach and do it all again. There were various left-arm exercises, too. Another was to sit on a seat and while steadying myself with my good right arm, put increasing weight on my left leg to haul myself up. At first I couldn't do it, and I was overwhelmed with despair, but I stuck at it and before long I was doing better. These were called 'sit-to-stands'.

For as long as I live I'll be grateful to Deanne, the head occupational therapist, and her colleague Rebecca. Rebecca took a particular interest in me and we were on the same wavelength.

When I got stronger, Rebecca would say, 'John, I want you to do a hundred sit-to-stands.' I'd say, 'Rebecca, I'll do a hundred and seven.' And I bloody-well would. I wanted to get out of that hospital and I could only achieve that, as I'd achieved everything else in my life, by putting in the hard work – and I also wanted to please Rebecca.

By lunchtime, after two hours of rehab therapy, I'd be tired and go back to my bed for a rest before returning to my exercises at 2.30 pm. Lying there in bed I'd think, 'Oh you beaut, I'm going to have a little snooze.' I'd go to sleep, but every day, right on 2.30 pm Rebecca would come to fetch me. She'd often have to wake me, and she'd do that by tickling my left foot. At first I couldn't feel anything because that was my bad foot. After a while I could feel a faint touch and would wake up.

After my daily session I'd shower, and even that presented problems. After a stroke your body can be extra-sensitive to temperature. Warm water can feel like it's boiling; cool water can feel freezing. So it was important that the shower water was lukewarm.

Rehab wasn't easy. It was gruelling and it hurt. Improvement was slow and only achieved after enormous effort and dedication. I often felt humiliated and angry that this body of mine that had served me so well had let me down. I had to fight hard against feelings of self-pity that threatened to engulf me at times. This, I'm told, is pretty normal for stroke victims. When things got tough I'd remember what Dad used to say when I was feeling down in the dumps: 'Never complain, John, there's always someone worse off than you.' That inspired me to tell myself: 'This bloody stroke won't beat me. It won't!'

Getting Better, Slowly

Typically, I set myself a goal. I reckoned it would take me forty months to overcome the stroke, and another forty months to return to good shape. That amounted to a bit more than six-and-a-half years.

Every time someone from my ward went home I promised myself that I'd be out of the hospital soon as well. I'd ask the doc, 'When am I getting out?' And he'd say, 'We'll see how you're going next month.' Winter turned to spring.

After a few months I kept carping at the nurses that surely I could continue my rehab from my home. They said they'd tell me when I could leave the hospital and the rehab sessions.

I was getting better all the time. It was a huge accomplishment the day I managed to climb the ten steps of a little ladder designed to strengthen my leg. Step by step, while holding on to a rail and

Rebecca, I dragged myself up. 'Do ten steps, John,' said Rebecca 'Step up to heaven – if you come down before you get to the top you're going to hell. Ten steps and you can go back to bed.' Soon I was doing the ten steps, and then another ten, and another ten.

The thing about strokes is that you have to learn to do everything again from scratch. Because brain cells are destroyed by the stroke, simple activities we take for granted such as thinking, counting, planning, reading, speaking, eating with a knife and fork, comprehending information, understanding what someone is telling you, tying your shoelaces, has to be re-mastered. All of this is made much harder because your body is so weakened and you get terribly tired quickly.

Fortunately, because my stroke affected my left side and not my right, my speech and long-term memory weren't impaired. I had no trouble eating solid food. A lot of people who suffer strokes have trouble swallowing, and their plight is made worse because they have to have everything puréed, which eliminates certain nutritious foods that build up the body and help the immune system. As it happened, Peter Cruikshank gave me special treatment when I wheeled myself into his coffee shop, scattering his patrons, and yelling, 'Cruiky, a ham, cheese and tomato sandwich, toasted and cut into four with extra pepper – and a cup of tea. And have you got any of those caramel cheesecakes? Good, I'll have two.'

'Push Yourself'

I owe a huge debt to Peter's daughter Courtney as well. Courtney had been involved in an horrific car accident at the end of 1997. She suffered terrible injuries, including brain damage. We nearly lost her. But Courtney, thanks to sheer guts and the love of her family, fought her way back to health. Today she's been to university to study educational rehabilitation and works with handicapped kids, such as a little twelve-year-old who was permanently crippled in a car accident when he was eighteen months old. I was determined to make a similar comeback. Even though I was nearly forty years older than her, Courtney showed me no mercy. She was definitely into tough love. She'd come into my ward and make me do exercises: 'Lift that arm, John. Use it. Push yourself.'

It would have been easy to veg out in the hospital and not work hard at getting better, just lie in the sun on the veranda and lose myself in the TV programs. But I found myself doing little isometric exercises the whole time, in my bed, in the café. While watching TV, I'd work away, lifting my arm and leg. Like when I used to run round and round the oval long after my team-mates were in the showers, my solitary exercises became a point of honour with me. If I didn't do them I'd feel that I'd cheated myself.

A great breakthrough came on the day, three months after I was admitted to hospital, when Rebecca told me that we were going to start doing stairs – the stairs that led from one floor in the hospital to the next, five storeys of them. She gave me a carrot. 'John,' she said, 'the view from the top of the building looks out over Botany Bay, and it's just beautiful. What a wonderful reward when you make it up all five flights.' First time I tried I could only drag myself, with enormous difficulty, up three flights. I simply couldn't go any further. 'That'll do for today', Rebecca said. 'We'll try for five flights tomorrow. You'll make it.' I told her, 'I know I will.' And I did.

Venturing Out

After four months in the hospital I was well enough to start accepting some invitations to speak or at least make an appearance at clubs around Sydney. Fred Pagano, Bob McMillan, Graham Bowen, Amanda and Johanna would call for me, and load me and my wheelchair into a van and drive me to the venue. There, they'd carefully help me out, put me into my chair and help me into the club. Early on, I did little more than make an appearance, and break down when people clapped me for making the effort to turn up. After a little while I was able to string a few words together, thanking the people, and telling them a little about my medical progress. Then I felt up to making a bit of fun about my predicament. Soon the tears turned to laughter. 'Folks,' I said, 'the other night a nude woman patient came into my hospital ward. She must have been eighty if she was a day. She started doing high kicks right in front of my bed. She put the hard word on me. "John, super sex? Super sex?" I said, "Love, if I've got a choice, I'll have the soup."' I knew I was on the mend.

In late August I was taken to Parramatta Leagues Club to be present at a Legends of Parramatta dinner. When I was introduced from my wheelchair, the huge gathering stood and they clapped and clapped.

One night after my brother Geoff had driven me back to the hospital after a speaking engagement, we sat and talked for some time. I realised as we covered topic after topic, talked about life, sport and our childhoods, that it was the best conversation I'd ever had with him.

Peter Cruikshank was keen to take me on outings. Usually our destination was the pub. I'd have a secret beer, just one, and a bet, and a chat to my friends. First time, Peter asked Margaret if it was OK. My sister told him alcohol was definitely forbidden: 'Peter, he's had a brain injury!' But Peter knew better than the doctors, I reckon, and I'm sure that beer once a week did more good than harm. For me, life is about quality of life. I couldn't live if I was a vegetable banned from a few simple pleasures. I have a vivid memory of being in the front seat of Peter's car and only being able to read the right half of the numberplate of the other vehicles.

I started getting into the ear of other patients who were doing it tough. I tried to inspire them, as all my supporters had inspired me. I'd tell the people who gave the rehab therapy up after two hours that if they hung in there and did four hours a day they'd be out of the hospital twice as fast.

Hospital Diary

Johanna and Amanda kept a diary of the first months of my hospitalisation. It chronicles my daily struggle against my debilitating condition. Some days I won battles, others minor skirmishes. Some days I was defeated. Here are some excerpts:

> June 23: Dad had cornflakes and a cup of tea [for breakfast] but didn't feel like visitors or a shower ... I came to get him for his first shave and toilet – success with both. He slipped in the shower. Cliff Lyons visited ... Got the phone on and Dad tried to ring [a bookie] to place a bet.

> June 26: We've been asked to attend a conference for John's care as he's probably not going to rehab. Devastated. Peter

C[ruikshank] rang to organise a wheelchair. Dad enjoyed State of Origin but in bed at half-time. [Tried to serve his own dinner from tray then] had a laugh with nurses about the mess. No bleeding on brain, but blood pressure high; wanted to get details on clot in kidney.

June 27: Vision difficulties. [Many cards from well-wishers but] Dad can only read half of anything ... Told that we could help Dad with his reading by using a highlighter to draw a line down the left side of a page/column and reminding Dad to find the line before starting to read ... Nurse came in and spoke to us about strict visiting hours – that Dad got so many visitors and we need to stick to strict visiting hours. We agreed with her. Rebecca the physio wheeled Dad in and said that he went on the walking machine again and did well – better than on Friday. Dad wanted to sit in chair and not return to bed, and even suggested going to sit on the sunny balcony outside. Amanda and I got Dad into his wheelchair again, no problems. Dad did most of it himself ... I had a sneak peak at Dad's notes – considered a high risk for falls, mental test did very well and scored 28/30. Lost marks for spelling 'world' as 'dlrow'... Cliff Watson arrived at 4.45, after visiting hours. No problem for Cliff, and I gave him Dad's mobile number. John Gray rang.

July 8: I told Dad [that he'd been invited to a] speaking engagement on October 4, grand final day. He was very keen to go 'even if it's in a wheelchair because you've got to stay involved in the outside world' ... Rebecca says Dad improves each day but there's a long way to go. I left Dad with his visitor, Steve Edge.

July 14: Arrived at hospital around 11 am. Dad was reading Sunday papers. Aunty Di, Mum and Amanda got Dad ready for his first official outing, a local footy match. Was a chilly day so Dad was rugged up – singlet, T-shirt, vest, sloppy joe and his favourite Easts jacket. Dad was a little down. He likes the weekdays when he goes to rehab in the gym ... We all went down to the coffee shop and had lunch. Dad ordered his normal toasted ham, tomato and cheese sandwich (he said, 'Cruiky makes the best toasted sandwiches I have ever tasted') and two cups of tea. Within fifteen minutes we had taken up the whole shop – Mum, Johanna, Amanda, Di, Geoff, Rowena, Bob, Rhonda, Imi, Les Hayes, John Geraghty and Courtney!

July 15: Found Dad in the dining room rugged up. Looked exhausted. Allan helped us put Dad back to bed. Left him at 6.30 pm, dead to the world.'

July 16: Dad in good spirits. Said he'd walked by himself without his stick today ... Told his visitors, 'I'm just practising for the next forty years.' We asked the physio later about Dad's gym session. She said he did walk with the four-pronged stick with one physio. He is taking all his weight on his right leg but there has been improvement. The physio said, 'It's a step in the right direction.' More visitors arrived: John and Margaret Mayes, Billy Smith ...

July 17: Spent the morning at Dad's unit starting to clean up. Went to hospital at around 3. Keiran was visiting. Dad had a good physio session: some arm work – sliding a pair of socks over a board using his elbow ... Leg work ... the girls timed him over ten metres with a four-pronged stick. It took ninety seconds. Jo mentioned to Dad about living at her place. He was very happy with that – 'I'll pay top board!' Dad said he wants Mum to find him a villa around the Shire: 'Mum has the best idea about places.'

July 18: Spent the morning at Dad's unit, cleaning and clearing out his thousands of books, photos, tapes and videos … Arrived at the hospital about 2.45 … Dad wants to go back to the gym for another rehab session. He started by sitting on the bed and raising to a standing position. He did this in front of the mirror so that he can see how his weight is being distributed. He is still taking his weight on his right leg and finds it difficult to straighten his left leg. After fifteen of these, Kathy asked Dad to take a coloured cup from her hand and give it back to her in her other hand. This exercise is to strengthen his trunk muscles. His last exercise was to walk using the four-pronged stick. He went around ten metres. He is now able to swing his left leg through … At 6 pm Dad was in his bed. We noticed his left hand was swollen. He said he caught it in the bedside rails the night before.

July 19: Johanna and I spent the morning cleaning Dad's unit – windows, screens, kitchen, bathroom. We removed thirty-six hooks off the wall. What a nightmare! … Went to hospital around 3.30. Dad's hand still looks swollen – very sore … Dad had a beautiful lunch today. Greg took him to the [concrete] yard and the boys put on a barbie. Dad had a look at his truck and a chat to all the boys.

July 20: Dad had a few bets today, but lost … Amanda and Butts painted Dad's unit. Mum scrubbed the laundry and balcony. Imi and I cleaned mirrors and doors … everyone inspected the new villa. Thumbs up! We made an offer. The agent rang back and said no, but it may be negotiated.

July 24: Offer accepted on villa. Paid deposit.

On 22 November, five months and eleven days after I'd suffered my stroke, I was released from hospital.

CHAPTER 15

Love and Kindness

Sacrifices

Once I was out of the hospital I needed care. Chris used up all of her accumulated long-service leave to look after me. She'd been saving it up for years so she could take a well-earned overseas trip on turning sixty. When the doctor at last relented and gave me the green light to go home, he stipulated that I had to have three months with live-in care, in case I couldn't manage or had another stroke. Chris selflessly said, 'I'll do it.'

Back in July, Christine had told me she was going to sell my home unit. Hospitals won't let stroke victims leave until they have a carer and a suitable place to live. My apartment in Cronulla was twenty-eight steps up and anything but suitable.

When I got out of hospital I was still confined to a wheelchair for most of the day, and walking, when I was able, was incredibly difficult. Even today, nearly five years later, I still have a caliper on my left leg and need a stick to steady myself. Obviously I wouldn't be able to return there. Chris went to work. She sold the old unit and used the money to buy a townhouse just up The Kingsway, at Caringbah.

The townhouse, even though it was at ground level, needed a ton of work before I could live there. 'Perfect position, shocking condition,' Chris warned me, and she wasn't wrong. In fact, it was a shambles. The carpets had been destroyed by the previous tenants and the walls looked like Jackson Pollock had been scribbling all over them. And naturally there were none of the modifications, like rails to hang on to in the shower and by the loo, and wheelchair ramps, that I needed. I had no exercise bike, which would be a vital part of my at-home therapy, or gadgets in the kitchen that would enable me to cook food and make a hot drink.

The people from the hospital who came to inspect the townhouse weren't impressed. They didn't see how it could be adapted for my needs. My daughter Johanna was there and she told them, 'I give you my word it will all be shipshape, and very soon. Look, my father may not care if he lives in a dump, but Mother does. It'll be perfect.'

It was then, when I was making a new start, that I experienced kindness that makes me feel that I'm the luckiest man alive. Christine paid a thousand expenses, including the conveyancing costs. She gave me a kitchen and dining table, chairs and a lounge. She came around to cook for me.

I don't think there would be anybody in the world who would

do for an ex-husband what Christine has done for me. She and I had been separated for many years when I had my stroke. Life for us didn't pan out quite the way we had planned when we were married back in the '60s, but there is still a lot of love there, on both sides. If there was a victim of our break-up, it was Chris, but she is the one, more than anybody, who has kept my life together. No job or expense has been too much trouble for her. She has made her life hard to make mine easier. Yet if anyone was to say to her, 'Well done!' she'd reply, 'Oh, I haven't really done anything.' You have, Chris, you've saved my life.

Before we parted, Chris, our daughters and I were a tight family unit. Chris and I don't live together as man and wife, but my illness has turned us into a couple again.

The Kindness of Friends and Strangers

Chris, Johanna and Amanda and their husbands Ian and Robert, my siblings Margaret, Di and Geoff, Peter and Courtney Cruikshank, Graham Bowen and many others helped me financially and visited me all the time, often bringing delicious food. Courtney stayed with me when the occupational therapists visited to continue my rehab at home. Fred Pagano, a concreter, did essential work and put a non-slip surface on the floors. When he played rugby league for Newtown, Freddy averaged forty-six tackles a game, which made him a great favourite of Jack Gibson. Now he was putting himself on the line for me. The concrete was supplied by the company I delivered for. Steve Donnelly, a local carpet retailer, carpeted my townhouse for free. Bobby McMillan was a tower of strength. The bathroom was fitted out with new taps and sinks by

Enware, whose proprietors belong to the local Lions Club. Painters from the district painted all the walls and charged me not a cent. I'd spoken many times at the Lions Club, and never charged money because they do such a wonderful job for the community. Now I found myself the beneficiary of their good work as they bought and had installed the bathroom modifications, for free.

One day an electrician named Graham turned up out of the blue to lend a hand. He explained that years before, his mate's son had been seriously ill and they'd asked me to tell a few jokes at a small fundraising event they were holding at a Pizza Hut restaurant. He reminded me that when he asked me how much money I wanted to perform I told him, 'It'll cost you two slices of pizza.' He said doing all the electricals in my house was his way of saying thanks.

Men of League, a magnificent organisation founded by Ron Coote that cares for former rugby league players experiencing a rough trot (about which I'll go into more detail later), offered a strong helping hand.

Graham Bowen organised a series of fundraising events at Sutherland United Services Club, where he's the manager.

When the Roosters held a testimonial dinner to honour their stalwart forward Luke Ricketson, who had just overtaken Kevin Hastings' record for most club matches, his game jersey was auctioned. Roosters chief Nick Politis bought it for an incredible $18,000. Some $35,000 was raised for Luke that night. At the end of the evening, this young man donated the entire amount to a fund that had been set up for me. Luke came straight up to me and put the cheque in my hand. I was at Easts when Ricko began his long career there and I have always admired him as an ornament to the game on and off the field. Thanks for everything, Luke.

I had the most wonderful support system. All these people and plenty of others too numerous to mention. If it weren't for them, I wouldn't be here to tell the tale today. No question about that.

My Backyard Gets Blitzed

John Quayle is the former general manager of the NSW Rugby League and chief executive of the ARL and today works as an Olympic Games consultant offering advice to countries keen to follow the super-successful Sydney model he helped formulate. He and his wife, Diane, invited Christine and me and Christine's twin sister Diane and former rugby union and rugby league international John Ballesty and his wife, Robyn, to spend a few days at their beautiful property at Denman in the upper Hunter Valley north of Sydney. Of course we had a memorable time as the Canon spoiled us rotten, but unbeknown to me, there was an ulterior motive for the invitation. John had contacted the producers of the Nine Network's *Backyard Blitz* program, wondering whether they would secretly landscape my backyard. When Chris picked me up and drove me to Denman, the *Backyard Blitz* team moved in and set to work as the cameras rolled.

Prue Keen from Inside Out Urban Design created a blueprint for a stylish and accessible garden to suit my needs. It incorporated large concrete pavers on a single level so I could move in and out of the house, bench seating, a new fence with a barn door–style gate that would give me access to the adjoining footy oval, a new lawn and attractive but low-maintenance palms and ground plants to give me the peace of a garden without having to constantly tend it, which of course would be beyond me. After a Bobcat cleared the existing vegetation from the site and excavated for the paving and turfing, Jamie Durie, Scott Cam and their crew turned Prue's plan into reality. They paved and laid, Scott built and installed the new gate and a fence of treated pine posts, and Jamie constructed a barbecue of concrete bricks.

Meanwhile I was living the life of Riley up on John Quayle's postcard-perfect property. He has a nine-hole golf course and tennis court, not that I was able to use either! And a clubhouse done up like a church because his father was a minister. It has pews and a steeple, and on the walls is memorabilia from his football career, photos and jerseys, including his green-and-gold Australian jumper. In pride of place is a 'Simply the Best' poster signed 'To my darling Johnny, from Tina Turner'.

All the time I was wondering what the hell a group of blokes with TV cameras were doing there. They kept filming me, and I truly didn't have a clue what they were up to. I was out with John on his quad bike, and the cameramen were shooting us from a four-wheel drive. I asked John what was going on: if I knew I was going to be in a film I'd have dressed up and shaved! John told me to settle down, they were only up there making a documentary on the wine country. I believed him, not dreaming for a moment what was happening back home in my backyard. At the end of the day, we'd all sit on John's veranda sipping beers. I asked the cameramen if they enjoyed their job, and they assured me they did. Everyone up there knew what was going on, everyone but poor oblivious old me.

Backyard Blitz is an operation planned with military precision because the moment when the recipient of the new backyard arrives to find their home transformed must be shown live to air. It had to happen that I walked in my front door at exactly 7.25 pm on Sunday night so my surprise could be captured and beamed out to all the viewers.

Right after lunch I said, 'Righto, time to go', and got into the car so Chris could drive me back to Sydney. This was a potential disaster because if we had a reasonable run I'd get home at 6.30 or 7 and blow the whole party. Suddenly John Ballesty started to stall for time. He looked confused and said, 'Bomber, I'm not sure how to get back to the highway from here.'

'Well, follow us,' I replied.

Anyway, he followed us at a crawl, and that slowed us down. Finally we reached the highway and off we went.

We arrived home at exactly the right time. Chris said, 'You go inside. I'll be in shortly.' I did as I was told, still not suspecting a thing. I opened my front door.

'Surprise!'

I was stunned, totally dumbfounded, when everyone inside yelled out. The cameras recorded my shock, and my tears. All the TV people were there. The Ballestys and Quayles who'd got home before us. My closest friends. Old football mates, including most of the Parramatta side from 1977. Ray Price, Graham Olling, whom I'd not seen for decades, Ray Higgs, who came all the way from Longreach in Queensland.

Jamie Durie attempted to interview me, and I could barely speak. About the best I could manage, after I'd said how grateful I was, was to reel out an old joke. 'Jamie,' I began, 'like you, my father was in show business. He was a comedian. I was his first joke!'

CHAPTER 16

Men of League

The Brotherhood of Footballers

With the possible exception of boxing, there's no harder game than rugby league. It's a brutal and violent collision sport and for as long as those two teams are out there at each other's throat there can be no quarter given. And I have never known quarter to be asked. Men who play rugby league are genuine tough guys, it comes with the territory. Yet what many who wince at the body contact and the occasional blues do not realise is that an affection, though often grudging, is felt by league players for each other. Each player acknowledges that his colleagues and opponents have, like him, gone places where ordinary people never venture. They've played on while in agony from sprains and even breaks. A dislocated finger or shoulder? Shove it back in and play on. They've been knocked unconscious yet pulled themselves back to their feet and thrown themselves into the fray. They've endured painful rehab for their injuries, and gruelling training, sprinting up sandhills while their lungs burned and their legs screamed in pain.

Like old boxers, like old soldiers, there's a brotherhood, a mutual admiration society, of old footballers. Doesn't matter if they were deadly enemies on the field, or maybe because of that, the bond, one to another, endures a lifetime.

The support of old fellow footballers played a huge role in helping me survive my stroke. The boys rushed to my bedside and nothing was too much trouble. I was lucky because I always worked hard at being a mate and of course my media profile and public speaking ensured that people knew me. But sadly, most players don't stay in touch with each other after they retire from the game. They get on with their lives being husbands, providers, succeeding at their jobs. When in later life they hit tough times, as many do – because of old age, illness including chronic ailments caused by football, their failure to adapt to life away from fame, their enduring love of a beer (especially if they do what many footballers do and buy a pub) and a bet – they are often left to fend for themselves, alone. Sometimes, too, they have no dreams or goals. They come to think that their best times are all in the past. Goals, as I've said, are as vital as oxygen.

We all know tragic cases of former footy greats who are now always at the local club trading tales of past glories for beers.

These old footballers can be said to have fallen through the cracks.

Ron Coote's Vow

Ron Coote was one of the greatest footballers in history. A long-striding, hard-tackling, classical lock forward, his performances for South Sydney, Easts, New South Wales and Australia are legendary. But to me, the great triumph of Ron's life happened long after he retired as a player, when he founded Men of League. Speaking for myself, in the weeks, months and years since my stroke, it came to my aid and helped me through the darkest time of my life.

It all came about when Ron was visiting Milton Hospital on the south coast in 2002. A nurse approached him and asked, 'You used to play football, didn't you?' Ron replied he did and she said, 'I'd like to ask you a favour. There's a fellow here suffering the last stages of prostate cancer and he's having a very tough time. He's an old footy player, too. I think he'd like to see you.'

The nurse led Ron to the room of Doug McRitchie, who played centre for St George and Australia in the 1950s. They'd never met, but Doug had been one of Ron's boyhood heroes. He seemed pleased to see someone who remembered him. Someone with something in common, a kindred spirit. Ron sat and talked to Doug for some time, and Doug became very emotional. He was a man who was once famous and who now, forgotten by the public which once cheered for him, was facing a terrible battle on his own. After Ron shook hands with Doug and left, he got to thinking that there must be thousands of former rugby league players out there who've fallen through the cracks. Blokes who are sick or lonely and have lost contact. Ron arranged for other former players to visit Doug, and their visits made the old Saint's last months a little easier to bear.

Ron made a promise to himself that he'd never allow anything like what had happened to Doug McRitchie happen to other players again and he went to see his friends, former players Max Brown and Jim Hall, and they tossed around the idea of forming an organisation to care for blokes like Doug. There was some talk of calling it 'Dinosaurs of League', but Ron wanted none of that. Narelle, the wife of former Canterbury star and TV commentator Graeme Hughes had published a footy players' calendar called Men of League, and she was happy to let Ron use the name. It seemed right to him, a title befitting the new organisation. To raise a little money, a function was held at the New South Wales Leagues Club in June 2002. More than a hundred blokes paid ten dollars a head, and numbers were bolstered by a contingent of former Great Britain players led by the ex-Lions hooker Colin Clarke.

Men of League Are There to Help

Men of League's first meeting was held on 11 July 2002, again at the New South Wales Leagues Club. Some 140 players, officials and referees joined up to become the founding members. When I got out of hospital I was proud to be one of them. Ron was named president, and former player and past premier of New South Wales and retired Federal Government cabinet minister John Fahey agreed to be patron. Also on the board was Peter Simons, who had run companies in America for Kerry Packer and was a whiz at setting up organisational structure. He was named honorary secretary and worked for the organisation two days a week for the next three years and made sure that Men of League ran like clockwork on a day-to-day basis.

Ron then asked NRL chief executive officer David Gallop if he had any spare office space. Gallop let the organisation set up shop in an anteroom at league headquarters but soon, after Men of League proved itself to be well run and here to stay, Gallop gladly gave them an office at no charge.

Men of League Charter

1. The primary objective of the Men of League is to support former players, officials and referees who have fallen on hard times or for a variety of reasons have limited social contact.

The Men of League are there to help with:
- Medical operations
- Rehabilitation equipment
- Nursing home equipment
- Grants
- Counselling
- Social contact through visits, cards, and telephone calls.
- Promoting and supporting fundraising events for rugby league people in need of help.

2. To promote the game of Rugby League.

The Men of League are there to help with:
- Touring visits to country towns by a team of members with fund raising split between the Men of League, junior football and local charities
- The general goodwill achieved by reconnecting former players, officials and referees with rugby league
- Having the Men of League attend local rugby league events.

3. To offer a mentor program for players who have retired or are about to retire from the game.

The Men of League are there to help with:

- Industry network groups
- Information on job opportunities
- Job assessment and counselling advice
- Information and help from people who have had a similar experience of retiring from football.

No One Can Party Like Old Footy Players

A committee was formed and a fundraising ball was planned for the Wednesday night of grand final week in October 2002. I was kept up to speed from my hospital bed. The Men of League Ball was a black-tie affair attended by over 700 people. Thanks to ticket sales and auctions of a box at State of Origin, and wonderful media packages donated by the likes of News Limited, Radio 2GB, Big League and television stations that sold for big bucks, we raised $120,000. That was great, but our first objective that inaugural year was to make that ball a whole lot of fun. If people enjoyed themselves, they'd be long-term supporters of Men of League. I think a great time was had by all. No one can party like old footy players, and the night was made extra special when we honoured as greats of our game Jack Gibson, Ron Massey and Frank Hyde, and screened a video in tribute to the old players who'd passed away in the previous twelve months. I made a surprise appearance in my wheelchair and tears flowed, mine and my friends.

The ball is now a regular event, and each year we've honoured such legends as Kel O'Shea, Wally O'Connell, Harry Bath, Rex Mossop and Barry Muir.

Over the last few years Men of League has grown to have over 1300 members on its books, and now has branches in Brisbane, Illawarra and Tweed/Gold Coast. Further branches will be formed in the future.

The highlight of the Men of League balls so far was in 2005 when the twelve-year-old daughter of former St George and Penrith hooker Garry Longhurst stood up and sang the national anthem. Garry had tears in his eyes, as did the rest of us, when he thanked Men of League for giving him the chance to see his beloved daughter sing for 600 people. Then the MC, Graeme Hughes, presented Garry, who is suffering from motor neurone disease, with a wheelchair.

The Way We Work

All those former players who are doing it tough, or their loved ones, need do is contact Men of League and they can be assured of a sympathetic ear. Many hundreds have been helped. The kindnesses the organisation has performed are too many to mention and, besides, we don't like to grandstand or name the recipients, but here's a typical example of the way we work. A woman recently contacted Men of League from Caboolture, Queensland. Her 22-year-old son, a league player, was stricken with cancer and medical expenses were so heavy that she couldn't afford to drive all the way to Ipswich to buy food. We gave her food vouchers so she could save her money to pay for her son's treatment.

Men of League buys lots of wheelchairs, and then, should the user pass away, we give them to others in need. Nothing is too much trouble to repay in even a small way the blokes who have given us all so much. They should not be forgotten and left to fend for themselves when times are tough.

I think of my old friends who fell on hard times and passed away without support, such as Peter Jackson (who admittedly never put his hand up about his depression), and I think that maybe if Men of League had been in existence then, they might have lived. Who knows?

Harry and Cliffy

I'll do anything for Men of League. They helped me, so it's an honour and a privilege to help them. I've spoken at many of their functions, but usually I just turn up at every function to be in the friendly presence of my old mates. The late Harry Eden typified all that's good about rugby league men. He was one of Jack's favourite go-to guys. A small, wholehearted tackling machine with good speed for a forward. Harry lived not far from me, and was always there for me when I had my stroke, and until he died in December 2006, picked me up and drove me around. Harry, who was in his sixties, had been diagnosed with cancer but you'd never have known. I'd ring him up and ask how he was and he'd say, 'Good, mate.' That's all. Just 'Good, mate.' Other blokes would give you their complete medical history, but not Harry.

Cliffy Watson is another great man. He was a Londoner who'd never heard much about rugby league until he travelled to the north and got graded with St Helens and went on to be giant thorn in the side of Australian teams for years to come. He then teamed up with fellow Pom Tommy Bishop to give the Cronulla Sharks backbone in the early '70s and brought them very close to a grand final win.

Cliff was, and is, a rugged-looking bloke and a big hard man, a genuine tough nut, literally. Cliff had a hard head and didn't mind using it on an opponent. In the First Test of 1970, Australia vs Great Britain, a brawl erupted and Australian prop Jimmy Morgan headbutted Cliff. Jim gave it everything, ramming his noggin into Cliff's skull. Cliff didn't flinch, didn't react in any way, except to smile at Jim and say, "Ere, laaad. *This* is a Liverpool kiss!' And he let Jimmy have one of his specials, no doubt honed to perfection on the icy fields of northern England and the take-no-prisoners pubs of St Helens. He shattered Jim's face with his retaliatory headbutt, and the bone of Jim's nose was protruding from the skin. Afterwards, Jim's kids didn't recognise their dad with his radically rearranged features. You guessed it, Jim and Cliff shook hands afterwards and became great mates. They remained so until Jim died of a heart attack in 2006. Cliff was one of the chief mourners at his funeral. That's rugby league.

The rivalry against Great Britain was tremendous, and it was always on for young and old, but now we can't wait to have a beer with the Poms. Davey Bolton and Tommy Bishop both live in Australia and are big supporters of Men of League. Even current player Adrian Morley, when he was at the Roosters, came with me to a function at a golf club in the Sutherland Shire and got a big cheer.

Good Advice

When Men of League goes to the bush, whether in New South Wales or Queensland, it's assured of a top reception. They love their league out there and shower us with hospitality. They follow the NRL and turn up in their St George, Souths and Tigers jerseys. Graeme Langlands, John Raper, Reg Gasnier and I were guests of honour once in Moree, New South Wales, and there was nearly a riot when we did an autograph-signing session at the local Harvey Norman store. Beforehand I thought, 'This'll be easy. There'll only be a handful waiting for us.' But we couldn't even get into the joint, it was so packed, and this was a huge showroom.

It's always a joy to catch a lift with Cliff to Men of League functions. Often we'll go together out into the rural areas, and he is a wonderful yarn-spinner, telling stories of when Great Britain had the wood on Australia. Men of League would be lost without Cliff. Even so, he still can be an ornery bastard. He refuses to go on any trip where there's golf or horseracing on the agenda. 'I don't play golf,' he explains, 'and if I want to look at horses I'll go stand in a bloody paddock.'

Once when we were driving together somewhere out west I asked him, 'Cliffy, what sort of work did you do when you first came to live in Australia?'

He said, 'When I played for the Sharks I was a bouncer at the old workers' club down by the beach.'

'Did you get much trouble there, Cliffy?'

'Well,' he replied, 'there was a young drunk bloke playing up one night and I went over to him and I said, "Hey, you've got to go." And he said, "Why should I?" I said, "Because I told you to." He said, "What if I don't want to?" I said, "Listen, son, it took me eighteen years in the front row to get a head like this. I can give you one just like it in eighteen seconds, now PISS OFF!"'

CHAPTER 17

Kicking On

The Best Medicine

At the Men of League Ball in 2003, MC Graeme Hughes introduced me and called me onto the stage. My daughters wheeled me from my table, through the penguin-suited guests on this great night. To a person, they stood and clapped. When we reached the stage, Johanna and Amanda helped me slowly out of my chair, and then with their help and the aid of my walking stick, I slowly climbed the stairs onto the stage. The applause by now was deafening. Graeme took my elbow to lead me to the rostrum. I said, 'I'm right, mate', and threw that walking stick up into the air.

That was my way of saying I was still in there fighting.

Of course I still needed my stick. I need it today, years later. My left side is still crook, I wear a splint on my leg because the muscles have atrophied; I have specially made shoes, and my arm is pretty useless, though I'm working on it. I've lost half the vision in my left eye. All that aside, I'm doing fine.

I speak at functions around once a week, and invariably get a warm reception. I hope it's not because I've been ill. I like to think my jokes hold up. I've modified my act a bit, taking the piss out of myself and my disability. Well, you have to, don't you!

I even have a bit of fun with my slow-as-watching-the-grass-grow approach to the stage and laboured climbing of the steps up to the microphone. 'Folks,' I say, 'I'm sorry it's taken me so long to get up here. I'd have moved a bloody lot faster if John Hopoate was behind me!'

Laughter is the best medicine, that's my message when I speak these days.

Ladies and gentlemen, my long-term memory is as good as ever, although my short-term memory is not what it was before my stroke. I was walking down Oxford Street, Darlinghurst, the other night and the women of the night were working and I said, 'Hello ladies, how are you?'

They saw me tottering with my walking stick and said, 'How old are you, darling?'

I said, 'Oh, around sixty.'

They said, 'Oh, sweetie, you've had it.' To which I replied, 'Oh, have I? Then how much do I owe you?'

Anyway, I thought I might as well make small talk with them, so I said, 'Ladies, how much do you charge?'

They said, 'one hundred bucks.'

I said, 'A hundred bucks! You're putting me on!'

They said, 'Darling, if we've got to put you on that's another fifty bucks.'

The oldest of these women was seventy if she was a day. She said, 'Hey love, how would you like to come home and spend the night with me?'

I said, 'I've only got five dollars.'

She said, 'I've got change.'

Then I might say:

You know, folks, people are always looking at me these days and saying, 'Bad luck.' But the truth is my luck was lousy long before I had a stroke. Once I caught a cab home but when it was time to pay the driver, I put my hand in my pocket and discovered I'd lost my wallet. I'd have to do a runner. The taxi pulled up, I opened the door and took off down the street. This is how unlucky I am – the driver was a Kenyan!

Sometimes I send myself up and inject a little current affairs at the same time. At the height of the furore that followed the Cronulla riots in 2005 I told this one:

Folks, I'd be lying if I told you that being disabled hasn't affected my form in the sack. For a while there, female companionship was scarce. I have to confess I drove to a sex shop at Lakemba to buy a blow-up doll. I took it home and it mugged me.

I never stop searching for new jokes. It's become a quest for me. It's good to keep refreshing your act and, speaking as often as I do all over New South Wales and Queensland, I don't want to be accused of telling an audience a gag I told them last time I was in town. It's all about being alert. I find jokes in books and on the internet. Sometimes something in politics, sport or current affairs will strike a chord and I'll make up a joke about it. And everywhere I go, people tell me the latest. I picked this one up in the bush last year.

A missionary in the African jungle says to a Masai warrior in his best broken English, 'I teach you English.' Just then a bloke walks by and the missionary points to him and tells the Masai, 'That, man.'

The Masai repeats, 'Man.'

The missionary says, 'Very good.' The missionary indicates a river. 'That there, that river.'

The Masai warrior repeats, 'River.'

The missionary says, 'That good.'

Walking on through the jungle they encounter a fellow having sex with a woman behind a tree. The missionary blushes and stammers in embarrassment, 'That man, riding bike.'

The Masai takes out his assegai and sticks it straight through the fornicating fella's head. The missionary is appalled. He says, 'Why you do that?'

The Masai says, 'That my bike.

Back on Stage

In May 2006, I took the stage as Hoges (with Freddy Pagano playing Strop) at a fundraiser at Cronulla Leagues Club for Greg Pierce and Rick Bourke, two great Sharks of the '70s, who were both battling cancer. I was expecting it to be a hard gig. The month before I'd been a guest of Johnny Mayes at his beautiful home overlooking the valleys and the sea in the hills above Ballina on the New South Wales north coast and he told me, 'Our old mate has cancer of the thorax.' Rick had cancer of the brain, and his prognosis was not too flash either.

But on the day it wasn't hard at all. It was a joy to look down from the stage and see the faces of these two wonderful, brave champions, both stars of the 1973 grand final, creased with laughter, to see them momentarily forget their life-or-death struggle and lose themselves in a little good old ocker humour.

Typically, Greg, with whom I toured in the 1975 World Series campaign to Europe, donated half of his share of the money raised that day to Rick who, he said, had had to sell his home to afford the expensive treatment. Sadly, Rick passed away in late 2006.

Tommy Bishop got up and spoke, and so did John Raper and Rick's neurosurgeon Dr Charles Teo. Billy Smith did his usual trick and heckled from his seat, all in good fun. I followed the professional comedian Brian Doyle onto the stage. Brian is as good a comedian as there is in Australia today and, despite the sad occasion, he had the audience in stitches. Freddy and I went over well, too (even though he kept forgetting his lines!). Just being on the same bill as someone like Brian makes you lift your game.

A Changed Man

My life is not what it used to be. I'd be kidding myself to pretend that it is. Having a stroke has changed me in many ways. Doing even simple things, like having a shower, going to the loo, eating food, making a cup of tea or opening a beer, presents a challenge. I have to depend on friends to take me places, and I've always been an independent bloke. I walk with a stick. I'm on a disabled pension, which I gratefully accept, but I feel a bit uncomfortable because I've always been a bloke who has worked hard to earn money and pay my own way. Sometimes my frustration boils over, but not so much these days. I've accepted my situation and it's full steam ahead to get better, or as good as I can be.

My faith has become important to me. I've always believed, but battling a stroke gave me a new, clearer sense that we all need help from a higher power. I call it God. You might call it Fate, or Luck.

I'm sure there are other, maybe deeper, differences. For this book I asked three people who are very close to me to write about the ways in which I've changed since I fell ill.

My oldest friend, Keiran Speed, thinks surviving my stroke has made me a better person.

John's old attitude to putting in the hard work at training has come to the fore in his rehabilitation. He does his rehab and even goes to the gym, though I'm sure mainly for a perv! John says, 'Couldn't you cope with being a young bloke these days!'

I see him a bit and each time he has improved. If you'd seen him lying in intensive care, you'd never believe he could ever progress to where he is today ... But let's face it, his battle is far from over. His vision is not getting any better, nor his left arm.

It must be hard for a guy who was so into fitness and self-presentation to have his body let him down after all those years. I asked him the other day whether he is resentful that this thing has happened to him and he said, 'Look, if I thought about it, I would be. I don't think about it. I just get on with it.'

Thankfully, his body won't allow him to push himself to a ridiculous degree. He used to be a bit obsessed. He got into power lifting there for a while, which possibly caused him damage down the track. He was lifting huge weights and he knew all the weight-lifters and how much they could lift. He developed huge arms. He was always strong, but he got even stronger. I don't know whether John ever had regular check-ups. Because of what happened to him, I, and the other blokes in the surf club, regularly have stress tests, blood tests, colon tests, prostate cancer tests.

He's been overwhelmed by the kindness of his family and friends. It's made him a softer person.

My sister Margaret believes that since my stroke she has her brother back.

Before the stroke he would ring me maybe three times a year. Now we talk often. He'll call me three or more times a week just to say, 'How's it going?' So that's lovely. And there's more and better contact between John and Di and Geoff.

In Chris, my brother has seen the best of the human spirit, and now he realises it.

Except in those first few weeks after he was admitted to hospital, through all his ordeal, John has rarely been cross or depressed. He's a bit like me. When I was thirty-two I developed rheumatoid arthritis. I could hardly walk for about four or five years and was in constant pain. I never thought, 'Why me?' I thought, 'Why *not* me?' There are people dying in

Africa. There are people with no money. People who have no one to love them. Who have no family. I think, 'Why *shouldn't* I have a bit of bad luck?' A little bit of hardship doesn't hurt anyone. John, I believe, feels the same.

It was wonderful when Geoff came to the hospital to see John and they sat and talked like old friends.

I feel that family ties are very important and the thing about our family – and I hope I'll be able to continue to say this – is that everybody is willing to help each other out. So there was never any question about if Chris needed financial assistance after she and John broke up. Dad made sure that she got it. When they separated, it was quite a big change in circumstances for Christine. She had a tough time. Yet she has been so strong for John. She takes him to the doctor's, she makes sure he has his tablets. She bought a blackboard for his kitchen and on it she writes all his plans and appointments. Over the years I actually think that if a way could have been found for them to get back together, they would have. But, you know, pride or whatever got in the way. They still love each other.

John now is determined to give back some of the love and care that has been given to him. He wants to help others. In a way, he always has been generous. He was selfish and driven when younger, but never mean. When we were cleaning up John's unit while he was in hospital, we found so many letters from people saying, 'Oh John, I didn't mean you to send me a cheque, but thank you from the bottom of my heart' or 'It was so kind of you to visit my little boy in hospital, and thanks for the gift.'

Because he has lost some sight and is not up to cooking, my husband Peter and I go down to cook for him on Saturdays and his daughters and mates help out on other nights. One night we had spinach. John had some on his plate but he couldn't see it because it was out of his sight range, on the left-hand half of his plate. He looked at my plate and said to me, 'Margaret, that spinach of yours looks good, I'll have some of that.' And I said, 'John, you've got your own.' Another time we were all having lunch, sitting beside each other, and he started straight into my sandwiches because he couldn't see his own.

He is much more emotional … I don't think I ever saw him cry, but since his stroke I've seen him cry many times, and he'll unashamedly cry in public.

To Peter Cruikshank, I'm a different man and a better man.

Yes, he needs kindness and help, but Bomber has slowly become his own person again, without twenty-four/seven care which many stroke victims require. He can do his public speaking, come with us to the races and the footy, his great passions in life. John knows he's a lucky bastard.

He keeps telling me how since his stroke he appreciates a side of life he'd never seen. He had a charmed life, and now he has a fight on his hands. Now he recognises just how hard other people in this world are doing it, and he really cares. I like to think my daughter Courtney, who has recovered from a bad car accident, has helped instil this more compassionate attitude.

He also has a superb support system of like-minded friends. He's lucky he lives in the Sutherland Shire. There are a lot of current and former sportspeople living down here, and we've four surf clubs, the Cronulla Sharks rugby league team, the cricket, some fine clubs. A lot of people don't have many friends and when they get sick they've no one to help them through.

John believes that he got sick for a reason. After a life devoted to personal achievement, it was a call to him to put something back in the community. A lot of people come up against obstacles and don't think why they were put there. John's grasped that.

Not that he's boring. With John there's never a dull moment. Soon after he got out of hospital, Courtney and I took him up to our property at Wollombi, at the bottom end of the Hunter Valley. We have horses and cattle on 125 acres. One hot summer morning we went for a walk below the house, down by a creek. John was walking very slowly with his stick and his left arm was in a sling. Suddenly we realised he'd disappeared. We called his name, looked everywhere. No luck. Then Courtney found him. He'd fallen down and was lying there on his back in the blazing sun, unable to get up. In spite of his predicament, he had a big grin on his face as he lay there like a beetle unable to right itself. Later he said, 'You know, Cruiky, I love the bush more than you.' This is from a bloke who grew up in Rose Bay!

We usually went to the local pub at beer o'clock – 5 pm. One day John was waiting in the passenger's seat of my car an hour early. I said, 'But John, it's only 4.' He replied, 'But I'm extra thirsty today.'

Not a day goes by that John doesn't inspire me.

Do or Die

I still get a bit of dizziness, a bit of confusion. Reading is difficult, but I've set myself a target of a page a day using an apparatus that magnifies the words on the page that my blind spot prevents me from seeing. And I'm doing a new set of rehab exercises to strengthen my left side that I picked up at Lismore when I was up there recently with Monkey Mayes. Monkey is working at the Catholic college and one of his workmates who had a brain aneurism six years ago showed me the exercises he does. I do them every day now. I put my hand on a bar on the wall and lean forward and then push my body weight back with my left arm. It's like a standing press-up. There are exercises for my stomach, leg and shoulder. These exercises complement the ones I learned to do in rehab at Sutherland Hospital and the work I do on the exercise bike in my lounge room.

A good and endlessly patient friend named Greg Cummins takes me to the Fitness First gym in Caringbah. I perform simple, light exercise, including leg extensions, seated bench presses (the best perving spot in the gym!), straight arm pulls, squats with weights, tricep pushdowns, hack squats, the exercise bike and treadmill, arm and shoulder raises. I must look like a dickhead as I struggle with the machines, but people say they admire my effort. At least it's doing something. When I get dizzy, I stop immediately. And I have set myself the goal of mastering a different machine every week. People up there say, 'You're the most improved exerciser in the gym', and I reply, 'Well, I ought to be. I started with a stroke!' Greg, like Chris, has put his life on hold for me.

My family doctor, Phil Dwyer, makes sure I take it easy at the gym. He told me not to hold my breath when I was exercising, says to train within my limitations, walk briskly, get my heart rate up a little. Never overdo it.

I do a little bit of walking each day with my stick. I pound it out on the street and around the oval that adjoins my home. As I walk I keep reinforcing to myself, 'You will beat this stroke.'

Like at the gym, if I get tired or dizzy when walking, I stop. That day at the North Cronulla surf club gym I pushed myself and I paid dearly for it. I'll never subscribe to the theory of 'no pain no gain' ever again. And after my scare I make sure I have regular cholesterol and blood pressure checks.

I don't waste time any more. I appreciate every single minute of every day. I'll never take anything for granted again. Pigeons live in my backyard and I spoil them almost as much as I do my grandchildren, Tess, Imogen and Finn. The woman at the pet shop says I spend too much money on them. I reply, 'It's a special thing for me to just sit and watch them eating away.' And it really is. In past times if I'd heard anyone talking like that I'd have thought them insane. Simple pleasures.

I'll still have a few beers, though I've cut back, definitely. I eat well and heartily now. I've got a bit of softness around my belly that I've never had before. It's the natural result of being a relatively inactive sixty-something man. Gradually as my strength builds and I can jog slowly, I'll get rid of my gut. This disability will not stop me getting into shape again.

The Passing Parade

Life is a passing parade. Nothing is forever. My father died on 22 December 2005. He was ninety-seven. He was living in a nursing home and had lost a leg three years before.

Dad was a real character with a great sense of humour. It was different to mine. He was always telling me hilarious jokes, but they didn't suit my style. My humour is laconic and laidback, his was quick and witty. When he was in the nursing home he was having trouble breathing and complained of his problem to my sister Margaret. She said, 'Well, Dad, you're ninety-four years of age. You're going to get a few problems. I'm sure it's nothing out of the ordinary. I'm afraid you're just going to have to put up with it.'

Finally, a specialist checked him out and found he had a mass of polyps in his nasal passage. No wonder he couldn't breathe! The doctor was astonished and professed that he'd never seen such a thing in his life. 'There's hardly any space at all for air to go through,' he told Margaret. 'Normally I'd check your father into hospital for an operation, but I'm worried that he might not survive the anaesthetic. After all, he is ninety-four.'

'Don't let that stop you,' Margaret replied. 'He's a tough old bugger.'

We went to see Dad in hospital after his operation and found him sitting up in bed with two black eyes, courtesy of the nasal surgery. His hair was all sticking up on one side. Margaret said, 'Gee, Dad, you look shocking.'

He said, 'You should see the other bloke.'

He never really got over losing Mum. He loved her dearly and there was a sadness about him after she'd gone. He remained independent, and even when he was ailing in the last years of his life, Dad preferred to be in a nursing home rather than impose by moving in with any of his children. He fished each day at Bondi, shot the breeze with his mates. There are worse ways to grow old.

His funeral was, if anything, a happy event. There were wonderful speeches at the wake, and they played the songs of his favourite singers, Al Jolson and Jimmy Durante. Keiran Speed told how Dad would always lecture him, 'Call me Jack, not Mr Peard', but Keiran had such respect for him he could never bring himself to address him informally. Keiran's father Ralph, in whose garage we worked out when we were kids, died shortly before Dad.

At Ralph's funeral I was first to the church because it's difficult for me to make my way in crowds these days. I was sitting all alone in a pew when Keiran came up and said, 'Thanks for coming. I know it's been an effort for you.' I said, 'Keiran, of course I was going to come.'

In the past year I've mourned the loss of four of my footballing contemporaries: Harry Eden, Rick Bourke, Steve Rogers and Robert Stone, the firebrand St George second-rower who scored that runaway try against us when the scrum wheeled in the 1977 grand final. Sad times.

The seemingly indestructible Jack Gibson today suffers from Parkinson's disease. He doesn't get out much any more, and has become forgetful. A few years back, Chris saw him walking his Alsatian dog and she swore that the dog was walking the once huge and imposing Jack. He dropped in at Mick Souter's house recently, having forgotten that Mick had moved away six months before ago.

I haven't seen Gibbo for a while, but on 27 February 2006 I rang him. His wife Judy answered. I said, 'Judy, it's John ... look, this is only a rough stab, but would it be Jack's birthday?' She said, 'Yes it is. He's seventy-eight today.' I asked how my old mentor was faring. She said, 'No good, John, but I'll tell him you rang.' I called Arthur Beetson and said, 'Mate, you'd better ring the coach, it's his birthday.'

Sometimes Jack remembers. A little while ago he sent me a piece of paper that read: 'Bathing beauties never die, they just wade away. Old gardeners never die, they just spade away. Old teachers never die, they just grade away. Old bricklayers never die, they just throw in the trowel. Old cardiologists never die, they just lose heart.' Another time this came in the mail: 'Even contemporary leaders should know nothing brings a team closer together or strengthens loyalty more than caring. Caring builds morale and breaks down internal competition. It promotes a feeling of belonging. It creates trust.' The great man is getting on but he'll keep surprising me for as long as he lives.

The indomitable Bunny Reilly is not too well these days, suffering kidney problems. Commentator Frank Hyde, the voice of rugby league through my youth and playing days, now in his nineties, has suffered a stroke and has cancer. Cliff Watson is off the hard booze. He told me: 'I used to drink a bottle of Scotch a day. I don't drink any more. My doctor said to me, "If you want to die, keep drinking your Scotch."'

The fearless Tommy Bishop, who tormented Australia's toughest men for a decade, is having problems with his eyes, but is still a cheery little bloke, always up to mischief. Cliffy's old sparring partner and lifelong friend Jimmy Morgan didn't make it. After a life of hard toil – he drove a concrete truck and owned and operated excavation equipment – Jimmy sold his home in Sydney and moved to the sun and sand of Main Beach in Queensland for a well-earned retirement. Shortly after, he was coming out of the surf, had a heart attack and died. Life's not fair.

Billy Smith, to everyone's amazement, is still going strong. His whole life has been a party. Even today, morning, afternoon or night, when I limp past the Caringbah Inn I'll hear a pounding on the window and look inside and there'll be Billy, yelling, 'Hey, Bomber! Get your arse in here and have a Bundy!'

Frank Hyde once bet that John Raper would never reach the age of forty. But Chook, another epic party-goer, who had a bad skin cancer scare a long while ago, is still in great form. He turned sixty-seven in 2006. I rang him and said, 'Happy birthday, old fella, it's Bomber. You've outlived Frank's prediction by twenty-seven years!' Chook was amazed. 'You're incredible! How did you remember?' I often have trouble remembering my own name, but I'm brilliant at birthdays and telephone numbers.

A Letter from Kim

Kim Mitric, the mother of the little footy-mad cancer sufferer Matthew, called me last year and asked would I be in the central coast soon. As it happened I had an upcoming speaking engagement at Toukley Bowling Club. 'I'd love to see you,' she said. 'I'll meet you in the foyer before you go on stage.'

On the day she was waiting for me. She told me that Matthew had died and she had a present for me. Kim then handed me Matthew's prized Bulldogs rugby league jersey. That jersey is among my most precious possessions, and reminds me every day of Matthew, and that no matter how much hard luck we think we're having, there's always someone, like Matt and Kim, who are doing it tougher.

Recently Kim sent me a letter … here is an edited version.

Dearest John,

I will never forget the first time we met you at Balmain Leagues Club at a fundraiser for children's cancer. You and Jo [Richards] came and introduced yourselves to Matthew and me, and we talked for a while. You and Matt talked football and you gave him a few tips. There was a sports auction that night and you so generously and kindly told Matt he could pick anything he liked (he did – a signed Parramatta football) and you bid successfully for it and gave it to him. Matt was thrilled. I remember leaving that night and Matt showed you his banana kick with the football and you told him it was excellent! He was so proud of himself. You also gave me what you had been paid to appear that night as a guest. We were overwhelmed by your gentle nature, kind heart, compassion and caring, and the fact you were able to look beyond Matt's cancer – always – and just treat him like a normal little man.

I thought I'd let you know what happened to Matt. In March 2001, he was in hospital for a couple of weeks with blood clots in his lungs. He was doing OK, and the day after he was discharged he suffered a massive haemorrhage in his chest. He lost thirty litres of blood and spent the next six weeks in the intensive care unit on life support. How he got through that, no one knows. He was cancer-free at this time and had just started school after four years. Two weeks after getting out of intensive care, he had a scan of his chest to see how he was progressing after his haemorrhage and they found two spots of cancer in his liver. He was booked for radiotherapy and one week later another scan was done and there were now about twenty spots in his liver.

By this time he had relapsed six times, and had had so much surgery, chemo and radiation that our only option was palliative care. The cancer spread so quickly, to his kidneys, spine, spinal cord and brain and he became paraplegic.

Ten weeks later we had to bury our beautiful boy. He was only eleven. He was so heroic and brave when he was dying and made sure we were OK. He never complained or asked for anything and was only worried about what we would do without him. Matt passed away peacefully on 30 December 2001, holding his dad's hand.

As you know, Matt adored his footy and his Bulldogs. I think he was their number one fan. Matthew's most treasured and special things were his Bulldogs jerseys. He was so proud of them, and everyone thought of him as a little Bulldog. We would be honoured to pass one of his Bulldogs jerseys on to you (signed as well!) as you were also very special to him.

Matt also loved that you would give him footy tips and encourage him to play. We hope each time you look at the jersey it will remind you of him, make you smile, and remember the time you spent with each other. Matthew would be thrilled to know you are one of the keepers of his jerseys. We know you will treasure it as he did.

We know your health has not been good and we have been kept up to date by the newspapers and TV. We were devastated when we heard you had had a stroke and know your recovery will be a very long journey. We know you are making progress and with your strength of character, your loving family and friends and the support and acceptance of help from all the people you have touched that your journey to recovery will be complete one day without too many crossroads along the way. Please know you are in our thoughts and our prayers.

Love always,
Kim Mitric

I'd been honoured many times for playing football, even receiving in 2002 an Australian Sports Medal from the Government for my services to rugby league. But it's by kindness, I'd come to learn, that we're truly measured, not by trophies.

Harry Takes Me to the Beach

One morning in 2005, Harry Eden dropped in to my place and said, 'Come on, Bomber, let's go down to Cronulla and have a swim.'

'Harry, I don't like the cold water.'

He said, 'It's summer, it's not cold.' I explained that it would feel freezing to me because I was taking warfarin, which thins your blood and makes you really feel the cold. Even sitting on a chair with an aluminium back feels like you're up against a block of ice.

Harry wouldn't take no for an answer, so down we went. He helped me get my clothes off on the sand, took my shoe and splint off, and then he carried me down the beach and into the water. 'Now duck under the wave,' he ordered, and I did. It was icy, but what a breakthrough! My first surf since the stroke.

I couldn't stand it for long, so Harry carried me back up the beach and helped me dress. He put my shoe back on and attached the splint. Then we had lunch at a little coffee shop on The Boulevard.

Later when I got home, I felt something odd in my shoe. When I took it off, I discovered that Harry had stuck two hundred dollars in there.

The Importance of Family and Friends

I've never had so many dinner parties and restaurant meals as I'm having since I had my brain attack. That's because I'm pretty much unable to cook anything, and friends and relatives visit to prepare my dinner each day or take me out. I look forward to Margaret and Peter coming on Saturdays. Peter is a terrific cook. He does a magnificent grilled salmon and we kick proceedings off with a dozen fat oysters each from a seafood shop he knows at Maroubra.

On Thursday nights, my mates Larry Gaffney and Johnny Chisholm come and whip up mashed potatoes and grill bangers on the barbecue that Jamie Durie built for me. In summer we sit outside and enjoy a glass of wine. More simple pleasures.

Chris is an angel. It's easy for me to forget things. Sometimes I get very tired and lie down on my bed, doze off and the day's gone. Chris rings every day, and nags me to do what I'm supposed to do: 'Don't forget to telephone pathology and tell them that you'll be away next Tuesday, and you have to make a new appointment for the following Tuesday ...' Or: 'Tell me what you need at the shops.'

I try to repay her. Recently I came into a bit of money, a small inheritance from Dad, and I had no hesitation in giving Chris half.

Jo Richards has been terrific, too. Recently she drove all the way down here from her home at Rose Bay and took me to a lunch with some football friends at the Clovelly Hotel, and then I stayed the night at her place, and next morning she drove me to four different places all over Sydney to pick up things.

The little tasks seem the hardest. Like putting on a T-shirt with one good arm after a shower. You've got to twist and turn and stick your hand up inside the shirt and try to drag it over your head, then one arm and then the other, and you're all wet and the T-shirt's not slipping on. It's so frustrating.

Courtney Cruickshank still comes around. Her father, Peter, will say, 'John wants to go out tonight, would you pop over and help him get dressed?' She'll help me pull my pants on or do my shoes up. Little things I have trouble with.

Grandkids keep me occupied. I spoil 'em rotten. They know I'm a soft touch and whenever they visit they leave with a stash of sweets. Every year, to mark my survival, I take Chris, my daughters and their husbands and their kids to a nice little restaurant, up the road. The kids are terrors. The restaurateur installed lovely new suede lounges last year and I'm afraid when we left after lunch they weren't looking so lovely. Each annual dinner signifies another year of survival.

Speaker in Demand

My appointment book is full. I receive lots of offers to talk and so long as it's humanly possible to get to the destination I accept every one with thanks. I won't accept payment, all I need is my expenses paid: transport and a hotel room if I have to stay overnight.

In February 2006 there was the fiftieth reunion of the Wests Club in Wollongong and I was invited with Darryl Brohman and Steve Roach to go and do a turn on stage. As usual, I waived my fee.

Not long ago I was invited to speak at a club in Tenterfield, and ended up doing four talks in one day. When I got up there the organisers said, 'Oh, there's another group who want to hear you ... and another.'

With hardly any notice, I spoke at Grandparents Day at the local primary school. Luckily I had a couple of school jokes up my sleeve ...

I had a stroke and I've got short-term memory loss but my long-term is brilliant. I can still remember when I was at school. I used to love a lot of subjects, but English was my bestest.

I got caught cheating in an exam. The headmaster told me, 'Peard, we have a suspicion you've copied your answers from another boy!'

'What gave you that idea, sir?'

He said, 'Were you sitting next to Smith?'

'Yes, sir.'

He said, 'For question number nine Smith answered, I don't know.' And you wrote, 'Neither do I.'

Thanks again, Brian Doyle.

The Tenterfield visit was typical of my trips to the bush. Nice people, passionate league supporters, all trying to show you a good time and impress you with their town. Sitting in the local pub yarning to these big, strong farmers with their calloused hands, hearing how demanding it is on the land these days and how they would never give up, was inspiring.

Tenterfield is the birthplace of our nation, where New South Wales premier Sir Henry Parkes delivered the pro-Federation speech in 1889. I was hustled onto a bus and found myself on a senior citizens' mystery tour of the local region. We had morning tea and lunch at wineries, and I saw the beautiful old town, the museum, the building where George Woolnough, Peter Allen's father and 'the Tenterfield Saddler', made his saddles, and the farms and roads of the region. A far cry from the boozy bus tours of my footy days, but I enjoyed every minute of it.

My Turn to Help

I believe in karma. I've been no saint in my life, and I've done many things I'm not proud of. If you charge me with being selfish and obsessed with succeeding, I'll plead guilty. But there have been times when someone's plight – like Matthew Mitric's – has moved me deeply, and I've done what I could to help them. Maybe the outpouring of affection for me from people after I'd had my stroke was a case of me receiving what I'd given.

After all the loving care I've received it would be unthinkable for me not to try to help others. I've a new empathy nowadays for people who I may not have given a second thought to in the past. People who are having trouble. When I hear someone with all their faculties functioning perfectly having a whinge, I'll think, 'Mate, you've got nothing to complain about!'

I support Men of League and I've joined the local Lions Club, both because they were so good to me and to give a bit back to the community. Every second Tuesday night, Freddy Pagano rings and says, 'Lions tonight.' Then, 'Anything you want? I'll come and fix you up with pants, T-shirt, shoes, socks …' Ronny Pearce, an old referee who's become a good mate, is another who drops everything to look after me.

Not long ago, after I'd addressed a gathering in Coffs Harbour, an elderly woman approached me. 'My name is Dot Duncan,' she said. 'You're so strong, standing up and speaking about your stroke. Can you come over and see my husband, Reece? He's had a stroke, and he's a strong bugger like you.'

Reece Duncan told me he was seventy-four and a 1952 Kangaroo who played for Manly and for Wests alongside the great Keith Holman and Frank Stanmore. 'Is Keith still alive?' he asked me.

'He is, but Frankie Stanmore is dead.'

He said sadly, 'Yes, I knew that.'

Reece walked with the aid of a frame, but I noticed he gripped the bar of the contraption tightly with both hands, his good and his bad. I put my hand over his bad one and said, 'Reece, it's good to see you using that hand. Every bit of work you give it makes it stronger.' Now I ring the Duncans every week. Reece is doing pretty well, all things considered.

I find it the best kind of therapy to talk to other stroke victims. Hopefully they get as much out of my visits as I do. Bruce 'Larpa' Stewart, the Roosters' dashing Aboriginal winger who burned up the Sydney Sports Ground in the '60s, has been crash-tackled by a bad stroke, and so has my old friend Jimmy Lewis. I regularly visit both blokes in hospital and perhaps they see me getting around a bit and think, 'I can do that, too.' I tell them never to give up, to fight every inch of the way to get well again.

It always comes down to defining, setting and attaining goals. Striving to achieve them gives you something to live for. It energises your mind and body. I tell others in my predicament, like Jimmy and Larpa, that it might take them six years, or seven, but they have to believe they'll be up and about again.

The Best of the Best

I've found there's no better way to spark a good argument among rugby league fans than to challenge your mates to name the best players they've ever seen or played with or against. Everyone has an opinion, and I'm about to give you mine. I know many will disagree with the players I've chosen in my four teams: A Team Chosen from the Best Players I've Ever Seen; A Team Chosen from the Best Players I Played With or Against; The Best Eastern Suburbs Team of My Era; and The Best Parramatta Team of My Era. (As I was the five-eighth in the Roosters and Eels sides right throughout my tenure at those clubs, I'll leave that position blank. You can fill it in as you wish.)

I know some people will be outraged that I can't find a place for the great Johnny Raper, Bob McCarthy, Ken Irvine, Andrew Johns or Wally Lewis in the starting line-up of the Best Players I've Ever Seen. Fans of these wonderful all-time greats of our game will no doubt want me admitted to a lunatic asylum, and I'll wear that; but in my humble opinion Ron Coote and the four great English stars of the 1950s and '60s – Billy Boston, Derek Turner, Alex Murphy – and Dave Bolton just shade them. Likewise, Barry Beath doesn't get too many mentions when the greatest players to have ever laced on a boot are recalled, but when playing with or against Barry, he was invariably rock-solid in defence and attack, enthusiastic, brave and had a huge heart and will to win, and he provided a platform for the superstars around him to perform. As Jack Gibson knew well, and I as came to know, every team needs champion blokes as well as champion players, and Barry was a beauty.

So, like it or lump it, here are my picks … And, as they say, no correspondence will be entered into!

A Team Chosen from the
Best Players I've Ever Seen

Fullback: Graeme Langlands
Wingers: Ed Lumsden, Billy Boston
Centres: Reg Gasnier, Mal Meninga
Five-eighth: Dave Bolton
Halfback: Alex Murphy
Lock: Ron Coote
Second-rowers: Derek Turner, Norm Provan
Props: Arthur Beetson, Glenn Lazarus
Hooker: Steve Walters

Bench: Andrew Johns, Wally Lewis,
John Raper, Bob McCarthy

A Team Chosen from the
Best Players I Played With or Against

Fullback: Graeme Langlands
Wingers: Ed Lumsden, Eric Grothe
Centres: Mick Cronin, Steve Rogers
Five-eighth: Bob Fulton
Halfback: Billy Smith
Lock: Ron Coote
Second-rowers: Ray Higgs, Bob McCarthy
Props: Arthur Beetson, John O'Neill
Hooker: Elwyn Walters

Bench: Barry Beath, Rod Reddy,
John Raper, Brian Clay

The Best Eastern Suburbs Team
of My Era

Fullback: Ian Schubert
Wingers: Bill Mullins, Jim Porter
Centres: Mark Harris, John Brass
Five-eighth:
Halfback: John Mayes
Lock: Ron Coote
Second-rowers: Barry Reilly, Kevin Stevens
Props: Arthur Beetson, Ken Jones
Hooker: Elwyn Walters

Bench: Laurie Freier, Ian Mackay,
Kevin Junee, Russell Fairfax

The Best Parramatta Team
of My Era

Fullback: Mark Levy
Wingers: Eric Grothe, Jim Porter
Centres: Mick Cronin, Ed Sulkowicz
Five-eighth:
Halfback: John Kolc
Lock: Ray Price
Second-rowers: Ray Higgs, Geoff Gerard
Props: Arthur Beetson, Bob O'Reilly
Hooker: Ron Hilditch

Bench: Steve Edge, Peter Wynn,
Graham Olling, Neville Glover

Fine Thanks Mate

Right now I have three goals. They are to walk without my stick. To be able to jog slowly. And to win the next Men of League 200-metre foot race. I'm serious. One of the highlights of Men of League's calendar is a race for members over 200 metres that they hold at their annual race day at Rosehill racetrack. The event is handicapped according to, well, the participants' handicaps. Harry Eden won it in 2005. I've let it be known that my aim is to win next time. I told the blokes I'll hop on one leg if I have to!

They know me well, so they're going to be worried by my challenge. He'll be thinking, 'That little bastard will be running around and around that oval out the back of his place, practising for the big race,'

Well, boys, I'm not up to running laps just yet. But I will be. See you at the starting line.

All About Stroke

The National Stroke Foundation is Australia's leading authority on stroke. Much of my understanding of what happened to me on 6–7 June 2002, and what has happened since, derives from the information disseminated by the Foundation. The following, reprinted with the permission of the National Stroke Foundation, is basic information about stroke, that I believe must be read by all Australians. Your life, or that of a loved one, may depend upon it. Forewarned is forearmed.

Stroke Facts

The disturbing reality of stroke:

- Stroke is the second single leading cause of death.
- Stroke is one of the biggest causes disability in Australia.
- Over 50,000 strokes occur in Australia every year, with a stroke occurring every ten minutes.
- Approximately 350,000 Australians who have suffered a stroke are living in the community.
- By the year 2017 an estimated 74,000 strokes will occur if we do not act now.
- Over 50 per cent of strokes are under the age of seventy-five years.
- Around 5 per cent of strokes are under the age of forty-five years.
- More women die of stroke than men.
- More women die each year from stroke than from breast cancer.
- Stroke costs Australia $1.3 billion each year.
- Stroke can be prevented.
- Stroke can be treated.

How Does Stroke Happen?

A stroke can happen in two main ways. Either there is a blood clot or plaque that blocks a blood vessel in the brain, or a blood vessel in the brain breaks or ruptures.

1. Blocked Artery (ischaemic)

A stroke that is caused by a blood clot is called an ischaemic stroke. In everyday life, blood clotting is beneficial. When you are bleeding from a wound, blood clots work to slow and eventually stop the bleeding. In the case of stroke, however, blood clots are dangerous because they can block arteries and cut off blood flow.

There are two ways an ischaemic stroke can occur ...

1.1 Embolic Stroke

If a blood clot forms somewhere in the body (usually the heart) it can travel through the bloodstream to your brain. Once in your brain, the clot travels to a blood vessel that's too small for it to pass through. It gets stuck there and stops blood from getting through. These kinds of strokes are called embolic strokes.

1.2 Thrombotic Stroke

As the blood flows through the arteries, it may leave behind cholesterol-laden 'plaques' that stick to the inner wall of the artery. Over time, these plaques can increase in size and narrow or block the artery and stop blood getting through. In the case of stroke, the plaques most often affect the major arteries in the neck taking blood to the brain. Strokes caused in this way are called thrombotic strokes.

2. Bleed in the brain (haemorrhagic)

Strokes caused by a break in the wall of a blood vessel in the brain are called haemorrhagic strokes. This causes blood to leak into the brain, again stopping the delivery of oxygen and nutrients. Haemorrhagic stroke can be caused by a number of disorders which affect the blood vessels, including long-standing high blood pressure and cerebral aneurysms.

An aneurysm is a weak or thin spot on a blood vessel wall. The weak spots that cause aneurysms are usually present at birth. Aneurysms develop over a number of years and usually don't cause detectable problems until they break. There are two types of haemorrhagic stroke:

- Subarachnoid
- Intracerebral

These two terms refer to areas of the brain where the stroke has occurred. In a subarachnoid haemorrhage, bleeding occurs under the thin, delicate membrane surrounding the brain. In an intracerebral haemorrhage, bleeding occurs within the brain itself.

Early Signs Of Stroke

As many stroke survivors can tell you, there are often early signs of stroke. The signs of both stroke and TIA may be any one, or a combination, of the following:

- Weakness or numbness or paralysis of the face, arm or leg on either or both sides of the body
- Difficulty speaking or understanding
- Dizziness, loss of balance or an unexplained fall

- Loss of vision, sudden blurred or decreased vision in one or both eyes
- Headache, usually severe and of abrupt onset or unexplained change in the pattern of headaches
- Difficulty swallowing.

Stroke is always a medical emergency. If you experience any of these symptoms yourself or recognise them in someone else, call 000 even if the symptoms last for only a short time.

The Fast Test

FAST is a simple way to test for stroke. FAST stands for Facial weakness, Arm weakness, Speech difficulty, Time to act.

Using the FAST test involves asking three simple questions:

Face – Can the person smile, has their mouth or eyes drooped?

Arms – Can the person raise both arms?

Speech – Can the person speak clearly and understand what you say?

Time – Act FAST and get medical attention.

Preventing Stroke

Stroke risk is influenced by a number of factors. Some of these stroke factors, such as age, gender and a family history of stroke, cannot be controlled.

However, there are a number of risk factors for stroke which you, as an individual, can control and in doing so help to reduce the chances of having a stroke.

You can reduce your risk of stroke by keeping your blood pressure low, quitting smoking, eating a healthy diet and being physically active. Stroke is also associated with diabetes and an irregular pulse.

Certainly the greatest prevention is to engage in a healthy lifestyle. However, sometimes surgery and medication may be necessary.

Stroke Prevention Through Surgery

The two carotid arteries are the main arteries in the neck carrying blood to the brain. They can become narrowed at a point in the neck by a build-up of cholesterol and other fatty material termed 'plaque'. If your carotid arteries have become partially blocked, resulting in reduced blood flow to the brain, you may be advised to have an operation called a carotid endarterectomy.

Carotid endarterectomy involves removing the plaque from the area of narrowing and opening the artery. This improves blood flow to the brain and lowers the risk of blood clots or pieces of plaque breaking off and blocking blood flow. It is useful for people who have severe, but not total, blockage of their carotid arteries. Sometimes both carotid arteries need surgery, but they are usually done one at a time, in separate operations.

Though the results are usually very good, the carotid endarterectomy operation itself carries with it a small risk of causing stroke. In expert surgical hands, however, the benefits from the surgery outweigh the risks. As with any major surgical procedure, carefully discuss the situation with your doctors before making a decision.

Stroke Prevention Through Medication

Some medical treatments can reduce the risk of blood clots happening or control your blood pressure. These are important in preventing another stroke. Your doctor will determine which drugs may be best for you and talk to you and your family about them.

You may be asked to take aspirin or warfarin. These drugs help thin the blood and lower your chances of having another stroke.

Your doctor might also ask you to take medications that lower your blood pressure or your cholesterol.

If your doctor prescribes medication, it is important to continue taking it unless your doctor tells you to stop. Your GP will monitor your medications when you leave the hospital.

Lifestyle Changes to Prevent Stroke

There are a number of risk factors that may increase your risk of stroke which you can control and in doing so can help reduce the chances of having a stroke.

Your overall lifestyle including diet and exercise will assist in maintaining your cholesterol, blood pressure, diabetes and weight, which can be contributing risk factors for stroke.

Eating a balanced diet is important in reducing your risk of stroke, especially one that is low in saturated fat and salt. Eating fresh fruit and vegetables is recommended and avoid processed or canned foods as they can be high in sodium/salt. It is always a good idea to check the sodium content on the list of ingredients on the label; it is recommended that low-salt foods contain levels of less than 120 mg/100 g.

Maintaining a healthy balance between exercise and food intake is important; this will also help to maintain a healthy body weight. People who participate in moderate activity are less likely to have a stroke. Try to build up to at least thirty minutes of moderate physical activity most days of the week. Talk to your doctor about an exercise program as people with high blood pressure should also avoid some types of exercises.

Risk Factors

Risk of stroke is influenced by a number of factors, some of which cannot be controlled. These may include:

- Age
- Gender
- A family history of stroke.

The more risk factors you have, the higher your chances of having a stroke. However, there are a number of risk factors for stroke you can control and in doing so can help reduce the chances of having a stroke.

Transient Ischaemic Attack (TIA)

TIA, or mini-stroke, is a warning that a future stroke may be imminent. Early identification of symptoms and treatment by your doctor greatly reduces the chances of a major stroke.

High Blood Pressure

High blood pressure, medically known as hypertension, is the most important known risk factor for stroke. High blood pressure can result in damage to blood vessel walls eventually leading to a stroke. You can control your blood pressure by changing your diet and lifestyle, particularly through regular exercise and maintaining a healthy weight, or your doctor may prescribe medication. Normal blood pressure is around 120/80; if your blood pressure is consistently over 140/90 you have high blood pressure. The lower your blood pressure, the lower your risk of stroke.

Cigarette Smoking

Smoking can increase your risk of stroke by increasing blood pressure and reducing oxygen in the blood. Seek advice on how you can quit smoking as soon as possible by calling the QUIT line on 13 18 48.

High Cholesterol Level

High cholesterol level is a contributing factor to blood vessel disease, which often leads to stroke. To reduce cholesterol in your blood, eat foods low in saturated fat. Choose lean meats and low-fat dairy products; limit your intake of eggs. Your doctor may prescribe medication to lower your cholesterol but diet changes and exercise are still important.

Poor Diet and Lack of Exercise

Being inactive, overweight or both can increase your risk of high blood pressure, high blood cholesterol, diabetes, heart disease and stroke. A balanced diet eating fresh foods where possible is recommended. It is also important to maintain a balance between exercise and food intake; this helps to maintain a healthy body weight. People who participate in moderate activity are less likely to have a stroke. Try to build up to at least thirty minutes of moderate physical activity most days of the week. Talk to your doctor about an exercise program as people with high blood pressure should avoid some types of exercises.

Obesity

Being overweight or obese can increase the risk of stroke. Too much body fat can contribute to high blood pressure, high cholesterol and can lead to heart disease and Type 2 diabetes. If you are unable to maintain your weight within recommended levels, ask a doctor or nutritionist for help.

Diabetes

Diabetes, Type 1 (usually occurs from a young age and is treated with insulin injections) or Type 2 (usually occurs from thirty years onwards and is treated with either tablets or in some cases insulin) can damage the entire circulatory system and is a risk factor for stroke. Talk to your doctor about controlling diabetes if you are diabetic.

Alcohol

Your risk of stroke can be reduced with moderate alcohol intake (one to two glasses a day). However, excessive amounts of alcohol can raise blood pressure and increase your risk of stroke.

Irregular Pulse (Atrial Fibrillation)

You are more at risk of stroke if you have an irregular pulse due to the condition atrial fibrillation or AF. Your doctor can diagnose this condition and advise you on how best to manage this if it happens. If you experience symptoms such as palpitations, weakness, faintness or breathlessness, it is important to see a doctor for diagnosis and treatment.

Recovering From Stroke

What happens for people after a stroke is different for everybody. It depends on what sort of stroke a person has had and where in the brain the stroke has happened.

Different people will recover in different ways. Generally, most of the recovery takes place in the first six months after a stroke. However, people can keep improving for many years. For many people, they get better as they get used to living with the changes that have happened after the stroke.

The care that people get after stroke is also different. Some people will be cared for in a hospital and go to another hospital for rehabilitation. Some people will go home after a very short period of time, while others may need months of rehabilitation.

When someone has a stroke, the doctors and the team will need to work out what has happened (diagnosis). Then the team works with the person and his or her family to make sure the best recovery happens. The team will also make sure that each stroke survivor is able to get the support he or she needs at home.

When people go home after a stroke it can take some time to get used to the changes that have happened. This might be changes to how the person can move or talk. It might be changes with work or hobbies. There are support services for stroke survivors when they go home. These make it easier to get used to life after stroke.

Life After Stroke

When you first go home after a stroke your family and friends will be your most valuable support. It is important, as much as possible, to get back to the life you enjoyed before your stroke. There are a number of stroke support groups and carer groups, which you and your family may wish to contact.

After a stroke, both the stroke survivor and the family are often frightened about being at home again and getting used to life after stroke. Carers might be worried about leaving the stroke survivor at home alone or about the possibility of another stroke. If you have any questions and fears about being at home, talk to your doctor and the stroke team.

Life after stroke has its own particular challenges that will take time, support and determination to adjust to. A stroke survivor has to get used to doing things differently and it can impact on intimacy, relationships and on work and hobbies. Help might be provided by your GP, by family or friends, from other stroke survivors of through organisations like the National Stroke Foundation.

What Is strokesafe™?

strokesafe™ is an important public health campaign, run by the National Stroke Foundation, that aims to teach Australians how to make themselves safe from stroke. Over the next ten years we aim to save 110,000 Australians from stroke.

Stroke is Australia's second biggest killer. If something isn't done about stroke now, the number of strokes each year will climb from 53,000 to over 70,000 in the year 2017.

Contact Details

National Stroke Foundation

Address: Level 8, 99 Queen Street, Melbourne Vic 3000

Phone: (03) 9670 1000

Fax: (03) 9670 9300

Information line: 1800 787 653

Website: www.strokefoundation.com.au

The Bomber

* Junior Club: Bondi United

* Represented Eastern Suburbs Presidents Cup side in 1964.

* Played Third Grade for Eastern Suburbs in 1965.

FIRST GRADE MATCHES

Year	Club	Matches	Tries	Goals	FG	Points
1966	Eastern Suburbs	3	0	0	0	0
1967	Eastern Suburbs	0*				
1968	Eastern Suburbs	18	4	1	0	14
1969	Eastern Suburbs	9	0	0	0	0
1970	Eastern Suburbs	21	4	9	0	30
1971	Eastern Suburbs	8	3	0	0	9
1972	St George	2	0	0	1	1
1973	St George	15	3	0	0	9
1974	Eastern Suburbs	21	5	8	0	31
1975	Eastern Suburbs	24	1	18	0	39
1976	Parramatta	24	9	62	0	151
1977	Parramatta	21	5	0	0	15
1978	Parramatta	13	2	0	0	6
TOTAL		**179**	**36**	**98**	**1**	**305**

*Missed the entire 1967 season after being floored by hepatitis and glandular fever.

REPRESENTATIVE MATCHES

		T	G	FG	PTS
SYDNEY COLTS					
1970	vs Great Britain at SCG	0	0	1	2
SYDNEY SECONDS					
1968	vs Country Seconds at SCG (replacement)	0	0	0	0
1976	vs Country Seconds at SCG	1	8	0	19
SYDNEY FIRSTS					
1976	vs Country Firsts at SCG (replacement)	0	0	0	0
1977	vs City Firsts at SCG	1	0	0	3
NEW SOUTH WALES					
1976	vs Queensland at SCG	0	0	0	0
1976	vs Queensland at Lang Park	0	1	0	2
1977	vs Queensland at Lang Park	0	0	0	0
1977	vs Queensland at Lang Park	0	0	0	0

	T	G	FG	PTS
AUSTRALIA				
(World Series)				
1975 vs New Zealand in Auckland	0	0	0	0
1975 vs Wales in Swansea	1	0	0	3
1975 vs France in Perpignan	1	0	0	3
1975 vs England in Wigan	0	0	0	0
(World Series)				
1977 vs New Zealand in Auckland	1	0	0	3
1977 vs France in Sydney	0	0	0	0
1977 vs Great Britain in Brisbane	0	0	0	0
1977 vs Great Britain in Sydney	0	0	0	0
OTHER TOUR MATCHES				
1975 vs Auckland in Auckland	0	0	0	0
1975 vs Rouergue in Albi	0	0	0	0
1975 vs England in Leeds	1	0	0	3

	Matches	Tries	Goals	FG	Points
GRAND TOTAL:	**199**	**42**	**107**	**2**	**343**

COACHING RECORD

FIRST GRADE CLUB LEVEL

1980	Parramatta	(Played 22 games, Won 11, Drew 2, Lost 9)
1982	Penrith	(Played 26 games, Won 7, Drew 1, Lost 18)
1983	Penrith	(Played 26 games, Won 9, Lost 17)

REPRESENTATIVE

1987	City Firsts	Won 52-12
1988	City Origin	Won 20-18
1988	New South Wales	State of Origin (Played 3, Lost 3)
1989	City Firsts	Won 18-10
1990	City Firsts	Won 38-26

FG = Field Goal.

A NOTE ON SOURCES

The material in this book is based on an extensive series of interviews conducted over fourteen months with John Peard, his family and friends ...

The publishers are immensely grateful to John's sister Margaret Moscatt for speaking long and generously about John's parents, family, youth and life away from football, and especially the events surrounding his stroke, and for making available the Peard family albums. Thanks too to Peter Moscatt, Geoff Peard, Keiran Speed, Peter Cruikshank and Greg Cummins for their memories and insights. John's daughters Amanda and Johanna allowed access to their diaries kept while John was recovering from stroke. For football and stroke recovery recollections, thanks to John Quayle, Ian Heads, Ron Massey, John Mayes, Arthur Beetson, Ron Coote and Gary Lester. Kim Mitric graciously granted permission to quote from her letter to John concerning her son Matthew.

Special thanks to Ron Coote and Martin Cook at Men of League for explaining the goals and achievements of this marvellous organisation, and to the Australian Stroke Foundation for supplying details about stroke, its prevalence in Australia, and for vetting the manuscript.

And to the great comedians whose jokes and yarns John has enjoyed and been inspired by: Brian Doyle, Kevin 'Bloody' Wilson, Danny McMaster, Ray Seagar, Col Reilly, Johnny Garfield, Bill Cosby and Paul Hogan.

The following books and magazines provided valuable background: *Big Artie: The Autobiography*, by Arthur Beetson with Ian Heads (ABC Books); *Played Strong, Done Fine*, by Jack Gibson with Ian Heads (Ironbark Press); *Winning Starts On Monday*, by Jack Gibson with Ian Heads (Ironbark Press); *Never Before, Never Again: The Rugby League Miracle at St George and The Lives of the Great Saints Since*, by Larry Writer (Macmillan); *True Blue: The Story of the NSW Rugby League*, by Ian Heads (Ironbark Press); *The Story of Australian Rugby League*, by Gary Lester (Lester-Townsend Publishing).

No-One's Indestructible: Surviving Strokes and Avoiding Them, by John Newcombe (Pan); *My Year Off: Rediscovering Life After a Stroke*, by Robert McCrum (Picador); *My Stroke of Luck*, by Kirk Douglas (HarperPerennial); *Five Pillars of Leadership*, by Paul J Meyer (Insight Publishing Group); *24 Keys That Bring Complete Success: Fortune, Family, Faith*, by Paul J Meyer (Bridge Logos Publishers); *The Lombardi Rules*, by Vince Lombardi (McGraw-Hill); *Run To Win: Vince Lombardi on Coaching and Leadership*, by Donald T Phillips (St Martin's Griffin); *Rugby League Week, Rugby League News, The Daily Telegraph, The Sydney Morning Herald, The Daily Mirror* and in *The Sun*.

www.ingramcontent.com/pod-product-compliance
Lightning Source LLC
Chambersburg PA
CBHW032117020426
42334CB00016B/987